THE
SLOW BURN
FITNESS REVOLUTION

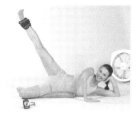

THE
SLOW BURN
FITNESS REVOLUTION

Get the Body You Want

in Just

30 Minutes a Week

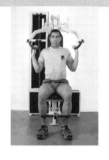

Fredrick Hahn, Michael R. Eades, M.D.,
and Mary Dan Eades, M.D.

Photographs by Marc Witz

C

Century · London

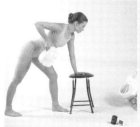

Published by Century in 2003

1 3 5 7 9 10 8 6 4 2

First published in the US by Broadway Books, a division of Random House Inc.

First published in the United Kingdom in 2003 by Century
The Random House Group Limited
20 Vauxhall Bridge Road, London SW1V 2SA

Random House Australia (Pty) Limited
20 Alfred Street, Milsons Point, Sydney,
New South Wales 2061, Australia

Random House New Zealand Limited
18 Poland Road, Glenfield
Auckland 10, New Zealand

Random House South Africa (Pty) Limited
Endulini, 5a Jubilee Road, Parktown 2193, South Africa

The Random House House Group Limited Reg. No. 954009

www.randomhouse.co.uk

A CIP catalogue record for this book
is available from the British Library

Papers used by Random House UK are
natural, recyclable products made from wood grown in
sustainable forests. The manufacturing processes conform to
the environmental regulations of the country of origin

ISBN 1-844 13186 6

Printed and bound in Great Britain by Scotprint, Haddington, Scotland

You've got to drive the body to the last inch of energy,
and then go on. You gain nothing by just going up
to where you are exhausted.

The body will only build and grow to fit the demands
which the mind makes. If all you do is exercise
until the body is tired, the body will get lazy
and stop a bit shorter every time.

You have to go to the point of exhaustion and go on.
That way, the body will figure out, "We've got to build up
more body strength if that crazy mind is going
to drive this hard."

If you always quit when you are merely tired,
you will not gain. Once you let the body tell
the mind when to quit, you are whipped for sure.
You cannot gain listening to the body.

We can become stronger. We only use about half the available strength of our bodies and less than that of our minds!

We can always take one more step! When we are on the
attack, we can always go one more mile.

—GENERAL GEORGE S. PATTON, JR.

This book is dedicated in loving memory
to my father, Victor Hahn.
—Fred Hahn

We dedicate this book to Rob Graham and Michael Shane,
who probably do a slow burn every time they think of us.
—The Eadeses

Contents

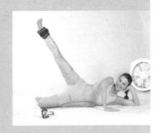

Part One

THE *SLOW BURN* FITNESS REVOLUTION

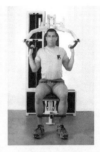

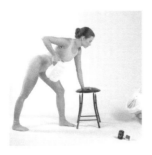

Introduction

This book, which combines medicine, exercise science, and weight training, is the result of a collaboration between a pair of physicians with a long history of nutritional and metabolic expertise and a strength-training expert who has spent years refining and improving upon the techniques of slow-speed strength training, which had their inception over twenty years ago.

If you are at all familiar with our previous books, the *New York Times* bestseller *Protein Power* (Bantam 1996) and *The Protein Power LifePlan* (Warner 2000), you may wonder why two doctors known primarily for their work in the dietary treatment of overweight and the metabolic syndrome would write a book about weight training. In fact, we've been touting the merits of weight training for many years.

Since the publication of our first book in 1986, we've been advocates of strength training as the hands-down best form of exercise for rehabilitating an out-of-shape metabolism or an overweight body. In fact, it was our advocacy of strength training in *Protein Power* that sparked the first blip of interest on Fred Hahn's radar screen and brought our work to his attention.

Since that time, Fred has become an advocate of *Protein*

Power eating as a means of helping restore the health of clients at his strength-training facility in New York City. The synergy created by combining his strength-building techniques with our nutritional advice has had far greater effects in restoring the health, strength, and vitality of his clients than either prescription alone. Amazed and delighted with the results he was seeing, Fred contacted us to arrange a speaking engagement at his facility. And that's how we came to meet Fred and ultimately to collaborate on this book.

In our time with him, we've come to understand that Fred Hahn is far more than a strength trainer to the stars on Manhattan's Upper West Side. He is an exercise professional with years of experience and training in physical therapy and rehabilitation who holds certifications in these areas, as well as in exercise, fitness, and slow-speed strength training. He's spent many years working hands on with his clients to refine his slow-speed strength program and has achieved the fastest, safest, most effective method of strength training we've ever seen. *The Slow Burn Fitness Revolution* is an outgrowth of this long commitment to excellence.

The Slow Burn method of strength training is unlike any you've tried previously. Paradoxically, it is both amazingly fast and very, very slow. Although you'll be able to complete a total-body strength-training session in under thirty minutes, you will learn to perform each exercise with exquisite slowness. This technique will take each muscle that is worked to a state of complete fatigue in just a few repetitions. Doing so sets off a cascade of metabolic changes that grow the muscles, strengthen the bones, signal the body to burn more fat, and increase the muscle's ability to draw oxygen from the blood, thus providing optimal cardiopulmonary fitness in addition to strength. When we first saw the method in action, we were fascinated.

For our part, we lay the scientific and medical groundwork of the system, explaining the "what"s and the "why"s in the first part of the book. In individual chapters, you'll learn more about what Slow Burn is and a bit about the science behind why this method works not just to make you stronger and build up your muscles and bones, but to improve your cardiovascular fitness, your endurance, your metabolic health, and your flexibility. Once you've learned the many benefits of doing Slow Burn, it's sure to become your exercise of choice, no matter what your current level of health and fitness is, and regardless of the goals you would like to achieve.

In Part Two, you'll learn the "how." We'll take you step by step through a Slow Burn workout, either at home or in a gym. You'll learn what equipment you'll need to do it on your own and get specific guidelines for doing each exercise in the regimen. For working in the gym, you'll find important do's and don'ts for each specific exercise and advice about using a trainer to assist you, if you wish.

Learning about Slow Burn will change the way you think of exercise forever. Once we began to uncover the medical and scientific bases for the many benefits of doing a Slow Burn workout, we were hooked. When we became convinced that you could honestly accomplish these kinds of health gains in just *thirty minutes a week*, we joined the Slow Burn Fitness Revolution. We think you should too.

The Exercise Myths

I get my exercise acting

as a pallbearer for my friends

who exercise. — CHAUNCY DEPEW

(American politician, died at age 94)

Three common myths about exercise pervade our culture today: any physical activity is exercise; all exercise is good for you; and being fitter means being healthier. As myths so often do, these three have taken on the mantle of absolute truth. A measure of the depth to which they have penetrated our collective consciousness is the way most people react to their even being called myths. Be honest. Weren't you just a little shocked when you read those initial statements? Sure you were—because if these are truly myths, then the implication is that exercise is *not* necessarily good for you. It would mean that the golf or tennis or rollerblading you've been doing isn't necessarily *exercise*, or that being fitter *doesn't* automatically make you healthier. And that's impossible . . . isn't it?

No. Simply put, some forms of exercise are good; some are not so good. And, as we'll explain, some can be downright dangerous to your long-term (and even to your short-term) health. Moreover, some activities that most of us would consider to be exercise don't give us nearly as much bang for our fitness buck as we've been led to believe: walking, for example. How can this be? The confusion arises out of common misconceptions about exactly what exercise is and what it isn't.

Many examples of what people consider exercise are in reality pleasurable leisure pursuits. That probably seems to be a nitpicky point, but it really isn't. Golf, softball, basketball, tennis, skiing, racquetball, and other sports activities are just that: sports. Games. Fun. There are undoubtedly some fitness benefits associated with these activities, but not as many as you might think. And—here's the kicker—these benefits come *at what risk*? Even golf, that most gentle of sports, sends its devotees to emergency rooms, physical therapists, orthopedists, and chiropractors in droves with hurt backs, twisted ankles, and injured shoulders. The other activities are even worse.

And what about the hard-core "getting-in-shape" endeavors—jogging, aerobics, roller-blading, cycling, stepper workouts, Tae Bo? Surely they improve fitness, don't they? Of course, but the way they do it is tremendously inefficient and comes with an almost harrowing amount of risk.

In 1999 alone weekend athletes and exercisers ended up in emergency rooms by the millions at a cost of some $22 billion. Most of these casualties were aging baby boomers injured trying desperately to stay in shape through jogging, biking, aerobics, roller-blading, and a host of other activities. Sadly, most of these sufferers probably accepted the idea that injury in some form—shinsplints, muscle strains, sprains, pulls, tears, or even worse—was the price of admission for better health and a trimmer, fitter physique.

Running is a case in point. Even if they don't suffer other injuries, runners end up with bad knees, damaged hips, and weak backs—all injuries that arise from the punishing beating the body takes when you run. It may surprise you to learn just how punishing it is, so let's take a look.

The impact transmitted through the ankles, legs, knees, and hips to the rest of the body from each running step is about three times your body weight. If your feet pound the ground eight hundred to a thousand times per mile, which is about average for the typical stride, and you are a 150-pound runner, you will jolt your body to the tune of about 120 tons of collective force per mile you run. If you are obese and trying to "get into shape" by running, these figures are much more frightening. A 220-pound jogger generates 175 tons of force. That's 350,000 pounds of force on knees, hips, and back. Brutal! If you don't think these forces injure runners, think again. Go pick up a copy of one of the many magazines devoted to running, and you're almost guaranteed to find at least one article on treating running injuries. Or better yet, go to the *Runner's World* website[1] and navigate to the sections on injury, where you will find descriptions of over fifty typical running-related injuries and their treatments. And as if all those injuries aren't bad enough, a recent study reported that runners and boxers had the same amount of a potentially harmful protein, S-100B, in their blood.[2] Elevated blood levels of this protein, which leaks from certain brain cells when they are traumatized, have been shown to correlate with neuropsychological deficits. So, not only does running pound your back, it pounds your head as well!

Legions of people are willing to accept these risks in an effort to improve their health. And why shouldn't they? It seems like every time you open a newspaper or turn on CNN you're being told of yet another study purporting to show

[1] www.runnersworld.com/home/

[2] M. Otto, et al. "Boxing and Running Lead to a Rise in Serum Levels of S-100B Protein." *International Journal of Sports Medicine* 21 (2000): 551–555.

the health and/or longevity benefits of moderate exercise. Despite the fact that these studies are virtually all flawed,[3] it seems as if physical activity *should be* good for you. To a great extent, it probably is, but not if you end up badly injured in the process. And not if you're spending hours and hours of your time engaged in pursuits you don't really enjoy in an effort to seize whatever benefit exercise has to offer. But take heart, there is a better, safer, more efficient way to reclaim or preserve your health, fitness, flexibility, and strength.

Slow Burn is a form of exercise that has been shown to provide all the benefits you seek from an exercise regimen in only thirty minutes per week, with negligible risk of injury. It's a revolutionary method of strength training that far exceeds the benefits of almost any other kind of exercise you can think of. Slow Burn will change the way you think about exercise forever. In fact, Slow Burn will establish a new paradigm for exercise, a whole new meaning for the word, and,

[3] A valid scientific study randomly divides evenly matched subjects into two groups: a study group and a control group. The study group is given the drug or prescribed the activity that is being studied; the control group is given a placebo or is instructed to do nothing. After a period of time the two groups are evaluated, and the difference between them is attributed to the drug or activity. Researchers studying longevity can't do it this way. Imagine the difficulty of randomly assigning people to two groups, then instructing one of the groups to pursue a course of moderate exercise for the rest of their lives and instructing the other group to do nothing. After all the subjects died, the researchers—if they were still living themselves—would presumably tabulate their longevity and determine if the group that exercised really did live longer on average. In reality, researchers doing longevity studies ask elderly people to estimate how much they have exercised over their lifetimes (dubious

like all truly revolutionary discoveries, a whole new vocabulary for talking about it. Exercise will never be the same again.

Exercise Versus Play

So that you'll know where Slow Burn fits in the universe of exercise and fitness activities, we need to define a few terms: *exercise*, for one. Most people seem to think of any physical activity they perform, from walking around the block to running a marathon, as exercise. By this common definition, bowling, golf, gardening, dancing, and even flying a kite are considered exercise, because doing any of them is more strenuous than sitting around watching television or reading. And it's true that these activities, undemanding though some of them are, all do improve fitness to some degree. So, exercise would appear to be any activity that improves fitness. But then, what is fitness? Well, fitness is what you get

---

data, at best), then wait for these subjects to die. The researchers then compare their ages at death to the amount of exercise the subjects reported performing and determine—typically—that those who exercised lived longer. Therefore, they report, exercise increases life span. These studies are flawed because all the subjects were self-selected. The researchers didn't randomize them into groups: the subjects put themselves into either the group that exercised or the one that didn't. Overall, the people in the group that exercised were probably more health conscious, watched what they ate, were concerned about their weight, and so on. So, in terms of establishing the effect of exercise on longevity, the study was worthless. It was as if the researchers took all the healthy people and put them in one group and all the unhealthy people in the other, and then "proved" that all the healthy people lived longer.

when you exercise—but that definition just brings us back full circle to where we started.

Let's agree instead that to be considered *exercise*, an activity must make you stronger, improve your cardiovascular system, help you lose excess body fat, improve your endurance, improve your flexibility, and build you up by preserving or increasing your bone density and muscle mass. Any activity that accomplishes all these objectives is *exercise;* anything that falls short, while perhaps beneficial to some degree, we'll categorize as *play,* if indeed it's a pleasurable pursuit, or *not worth the effort,* if it doesn't measure up and we don't enjoy it.

As you'll see in coming chapters, perhaps to your surprise, all these objective measures of fitness that we've said define exercise are chiefly manifestations of becoming stronger. The bottom line is that exercise is something that builds strength, and Slow Burn is the best way to do that.

You may think that all this business about what's exercise and what's fun is just semantics, but it isn't. It illustrates a point central to dispelling the myths of exercise. The distinction is evident not so much in relation to golf, softball, tennis, and other sports that you might honestly pursue for fun, but rather in relation to jogging, aerobics, stationary cycling, pumping a stepper, and a host of other mindless "fitness" activities that you might be doing, not particularly for fun but out of a desire to be more fit. We don't mean to imply that there aren't many people who truly enjoy jogging or biking, because obviously, some do; for these people, such activities clearly qualify as *fun.* What they don't qualify as, however, is *exercise* according to our definition. Let's examine why.

Virtually all the benefits that come from these activities derive from increased strength. If you're out of shape and you begin to jog, for example, you'll strengthen your thighs, calves, hips, and abdomen, but not the rest of your muscles and bones. The Slow Burn regimen strengthens these same muscles along with all the rest—to a much, much greater degree, and in about one-tenth the time. So if it's strength you're looking for as you grimly jog mile after mind-numbing mile three or four times a week to stay fit, why not save your ankles, hips, knees, and back and spend just thirty minutes a week doing Slow Burn instead? You'll be way ahead of the game. Not only will you get stronger faster and more safely, you'll also have the 3½ hours you saved to do something you truly enjoy.

In the same vein, if you're playing tennis, racquetball, basketball, or any other sport a couple of times a week just to stay in shape (or to get in shape) and not really for the enjoyment of the game, bag it; spend a fraction of that time doing Slow Burn (without risk of twisting an ankle or taking a racquet in the eye) and spend the rest of your time doing whatever it is you truly enjoy, which may not be an athletic activity at all. But if you do love the sport you play, your added strength and stamina from doing Slow Burn is sure to improve your level of performance.

But what about endurance? What about cardiovascular fitness? Surely we need to jog or walk or bike or do some other sort of endurance-oriented activity to keep our hearts and lungs fit, don't we? Again, the surprising answer is no. Although most people think of these two exercise objectives—cardiovascular fitness and endurance—as one and the same thing, in fact, they aren't. You'll learn why in Chapter 4, which is devoted entirely to the subject of strengthening the heart.

In that chapter, you will see that while jogging does indeed improve endurance, it does so not by improving the capacity of your heart or lungs, but by increasing your strength and making it easier to run. The more you jog, the stronger your running muscles become, and the easier it is to jog. Cardiovascular fitness is another matter. As the full Slow Burn story unfolds in successive chapters, you'll come to understand that what people commonly think of as cardiovascular fitness— i.e., endurance—improves as much with Slow Burn as it does with jogging. We're not saying that doing Slow Burn will increase your running endurance better than running itself will, but by the same token, neither will running increase your endurance for other activities—rowing, for instance. Your muscles must adapt to each specific demand placed on them. That said, however, Slow Burn will indeed make you a stronger runner if you run already, and it will make you a better rower if you row already. In short, it will make you better at any endeavor you're adapted to doing.

Don't Beat Yourself Up—Build Yourself Up

The promise of the Slow Burn fitness program is to quickly and efficiently build your strength without injury and without the risk that accompanies most of the activities all of us pursue in an effort to be fit. Remember: the goal of exercise is to build yourself up, not to beat yourself up. When you're stronger you can be better at whatever it is that you want to do, whether that means athletic endeavors, leisure pursuits, or simply everyday activities.

When you join the Slow Burn Fitness Revolution, your muscles and bones will become stronger, your endurance will improve, you'll enhance your flexibility, and you'll burn more body fat. Performing a Slow Burn workout will set in motion biochemical forces that will make you less hungry and get rid of many of the aches and pains that may have seemed to be an inescapable part of getting older. Slow Burn will definitely make you fitter and, to a certain extent, healthier. Why do we say "to a certain extent"? Isn't a fitter body a healthier body? Not necessarily, which leads to the last of the exercise myths: fitness equals health.

Fit Does Not Mean Healthy

To illustrate the fallacy of this myth, let's look at two examples. The first is that of Jim Fixx, the running guru and author who died from a heart attack while jogging at age fifty-two. Certainly he was fit. But was he healthy? His autopsy report said no. Fixx had a family history of heart disease and had developed coronary arteriosclerosis himself, but he ignored the warning signs of impending cardiac disaster, apparently feeling invincible because of his extraordinary fitness. Since taking up running years before, he had shed sixty pounds, run about 37,000 miles, and completed numerous marathons, and he continued to run fifty to sixty miles per week. He walked out of the house one day in July of 1984, began his jog, and fell over dead. With all the fitness in the world, he couldn't outrun his diseased coronary arteries. Fit, but still unhealthy.

Compare Jim Fixx to Sir Winston Churchill, who was not only obese, but smoked, overate, and drank with abandon, yet lived to be ninety-one. No one would describe Mr. Churchill as fit, but he was certainly healthy. Jim Fixx could have run circles around Churchill, but Churchill lived to be forty years older. Health is a state in which all the components of the body are functioning properly and there is an absence of disease. Fitness is the ability to perform strenuous work or exercise. Clearly, it is possible to be healthy without being fit and *vice versa*.

Why the distinction? Because it is important to realize the limitation of all forms of exercise, including strength training, when it comes to your health. If you have severe heart disease, following a Slow Burn regimen is not going to make your heart disease go away. In fact, just as with any form of exercise, it could actually cause you to exceed the capacity of your heart and develop problems. Slow Burn cannot cure cancer. These diseases involve health issues, not fitness issues. You can undoubtedly improve your fitness doing Slow Burn, but your health is another matter. For this reason, as with any exercise prescription, it is important that you seek the advice of a physician before beginning your Slow Burn regimen to ensure that your health will support your fitness efforts. While you are doing Slow Burn training, should you experience any worrisome symptoms, such as chest pain, shortness of breath, or headache, don't ignore them. Don't be like Jim Fixx. Seek the attention of a physician.

Even though exercise can't guarantee perfect health, it is true that you will improve your health as you progress with your Slow Burn training. You will strengthen your muscles and bones and improve your circulation, your sensitivity to insulin, and your blood sugar control. If you've got it to lose, you should even lose some excess body fat. But these are improvements in health that is already basically good. By engaging in exercise, you won't cure some underlying disease, but you will build upon and improve your existing health. You will become a stronger, healthier you in just thirty minutes a week. Now, instead of spending hours jogging, walking, or cranking out your three sets of twelve reps in the gym three to five times a week, you can spend just a half hour, or work out as little as once a week doing Slow Burn and take all those extra hours to the beach.

No matter what your starting condition is—even if you're currently quite frail and weak—as the weeks go by, you will become noticeably stronger and fitter. From your once-a-week Slow Burn session, you'll find all your physical pursuits becoming easier—whether that means playing a better game of tennis or climbing the stairs in your home more easily. Once you stop believing the myths of exercise, you can start working to build strength, and playing to have fun.

Slow-Speed
Strength Training

CHAPTER 2

Exercise and temperance can preserve
something of our early strength, even in
old age. — CICERO

Why Strength Train?

Most people think of strength training as something just for body builders and, absent any desire for a sculpted, rippling physique, not something of particular interest to the rest of us. But this common perception has recently begun to change. Lately, we've begun hearing about the importance of strength training, not just in building bigger, stronger muscles, but also in preventing certain diseases, notably osteoporosis. Today you'll see a larger number of women—even older ones—turning up in gyms, taking an interest in pumping iron to strengthen weak bones. But, as it turns out, preventing osteoporosis is but the tip of the iceberg when it comes to the health benefits that science now attributes to weight training.

Recent medical research has demonstrated that strength training is the most effective way to achieve a healthier and fitter body. And unlike other forms of exercise that can take their toll on knees, ankles, hips, and shoulders, weight work, properly done, strengthens the muscles, joints, bones, and connective tissues while improving your overall health. In other words, the goal (and result) of strength training is to build you up, not beat you up.

It's easy to understand how strength training makes you strong, but how does strength training make you healthy? At the most basic level, it does so by improving the metabolic health of your muscular system and, consequently, most of the other systems of the body. Let's take a look at why.

Collectively, the muscular system is the largest organ in the body, nourished and cleansed by the most extensive network of blood vessels. In fact, because the lion's share of your body's blood vessel (or vascular) system resides in your muscles, keeping your muscular system healthy of necessity enhances your vascular system. Contrary to common belief, most of your other organs, including the heart and lungs, exist to serve your muscular system. Improvements (or, for that matter, losses) here have an impact throughout your body.

The muscles you use when you exercise use the most blood, consume the most sugar and fat for fuel, produce the most heat, and require the most energy of all the body's systems. Not only is the muscular system the largest, most energy-consuming, heat-producing organ in the body, it's the only one whose function you can directly improve through exercise. There are no exercises you can do to improve your liver function or kidney function or your gastrointestinal tract function. And, although it may surprise you, there isn't much you can do to directly improve your heart and lung function. (As you'll learn in coming chapters, the perceived improvement in the heart and lungs that occurs with exercise is actually just an improvement in the muscles' ability to take up oxygen from the blood.) But all the body's organ systems do have one dreadful thing in common: they deteriorate with age. That's right, the older you get, the less efficiently your liver, kidneys, heart, lungs, and all the rest work. Even your muscular system deteriorates with age.

It's a sad but true fact of life that as you pass the age of twenty, you start losing a little bit of your muscle mass each year, not much at first, but more and more as you get older; between the ages of twenty and forty, in fact, total muscle mass can decrease by as much as 40 percent. This age-related decline occurs regardless of how active you are—unless, as you'll soon see, you regularly engage in a strength-building regimen that's properly done. (Surprisingly, studies have shown that both the sedentary and the physically active lose muscle tissue at about the same rate.) By the time you pass fifty, you're losing about 1 percent of your muscle mass each year. It's no wonder that you can't do what you could when you were younger; you simply don't have the same amount of muscle or strength that you did then. But you don't have to drift off into your dotage without a fight. You can maintain and even gain both muscle and strength despite the fact that—like everyone else—you're fighting the calendar. Studies have shown that the diminished strength that occurs with aging isn't an inevitable consequence of getting old: in both men and women of all ages, it's been shown repeatedly that strength is a function of muscle mass. And that's wonderful, because it means that if you can somehow restore the level of muscle mass you had at age twenty, you'll be just as strong as you were then—even if you're in your eighties. The good news is that you can do just that. Let's examine how.

Apart from eating a sound, nutritious diet devoid of toxic insults (such as excess sugar, fructose, and *trans* fats, the primary culprits in promoting diabetes, heart disease, and obesity) and not smoking or drinking to excess, there's not a lot that you can do directly to stop age-related decline in liver, kidney, heart, and lung function. The muscular system is another matter, and that's the big difference between it and these other organs: you can do something about muscle loss.

If you do the proper type of strength training, you can stop and even reverse the loss of muscle tissue. This, in turn, triggers a host of benefits in the body's other organ systems. To provide the increased muscle mass with fuel and nutrients, your liver begins to work more efficiently. Your fitter muscles, better able to extract oxygen from the blood, put less demand on your heart and lungs when you perform any type of physical work, and you find that you're no longer puffing, panting, and feeling your heart pound as you walk or climb stairs. So, by improving muscle strength and mass, which you can do directly with a properly performed strength-training program, you will indirectly improve the health of all the other systems in the body.

Why Join the Slow Burn Revolution?

Although it's true that conventional strength training—if it's properly done—can bring about gains in muscle, strength, and fitness, it can be both tedious and dangerous. Traditional body builders spend endless hours in the gym and often injure themselves pursuing their goal of lifting ever heavier weights through more reps. Like the jolt that jogging gives your knees, hips, and ankles, performing the usual three sets of eight to twelve repetitions puts tremendous repetitive strain on the tendons and ligaments that support and stabilize the joints. In traditional-style weight training, lifters use momentum and gravity to help them lift heavier weights and lift them faster, and to snap the weights back and forth; in doing so, they risk repetitive trauma to the joints, ligaments, and tendons. At the very least, the consequence of this incorrect sort of weight lifting is soreness, with the ever-present risk of overuse injuries, strained or torn muscles, and tendonitis. Acceptance of soreness and injury is showcased in the much-repeated weight lifter's mantra: No Pain, No Gain.

By contrast, Slow Burn takes a completely different approach to lifting weights, with an emphasis on the three most important aspects of a strength-training program: safety, effectiveness, and efficiency. Instead of spending hours in the gym grunting, sweating, and straining, you'll learn how to do a controlled Slow Burn that will improve your strength, rebuild your bones and muscles, restore your vitality, and postpone the aging process more safely and effectively than any other single form of exercise, in just thirty minutes a week. Sounds impossible, but it's absolutely true.

The secret to building strength quickly is exercising slowly and minimizing the effects of momentum and gravity. Although you can easily complete a full Slow Burn workout in under thirty minutes, you will perform each individual exercise with deliberate slowness. And while "slow" might sound easy, the focused slowness that eliminates momentum actually forces your muscles to work much harder. You can easily demonstrate the impact of reducing momentum. Get up right now and try performing a deep knee-bend the way you would normally do—go down quickly and bounce up. Now try doing it incredibly slowly—take ten seconds to go down and ten seconds to rise up. Performed slowly, it's a totally different exercise, isn't it? Without momentum to assist you, your muscles had to work much harder the second time.

And it's the elimination of momentum that's at the heart of the Slow Burn Revolution, producing maximal strength gains with a minimal time investment. Studies have shown that subjects following a slow-speed strength-training regimen achieve 50 to 100 percent greater strength gains than those in a traditional weight-lifting program. That's up to two times as much strength, doing many fewer reps, taking far less time, with much less risk of injury, and in many cases with much less weight. How can this be so? Let's take a look.

The Secret of the Big, Fast Burn

Exercise scientists have identified four different types of muscle fibers: slow-twitch fibers (the smallest ones), two types of intermediate-twitch fibers (slightly larger and slightly faster), and fast-twitch fibers (the biggest, fastest fibers of all).[1] The types differ not just in their size and the speed with which they can fire and contract, but in their use in the body. The big fast-twitch fibers, for instance, are designed for situations requiring explosive power of short duration. Large predators, lions for example, have great numbers of fast-twitch fibers in their muscles so they can muster the explosive speed and power necessary to bring down large prey. The slower fibers, while unable to generate the zero-to-sixty power of their bigger cousins, have the edge in endurance. Animals (including humans) who lope along at a slow, steady pace for mile after mile after mile have a preponderance of smaller, slower muscle fibers. To envision the difference, bring to mind the image of the marathon runner, or the giraffe gracefully ranging across the open savannah.

We all have some of each fiber type in our muscles, al-

[1]Exercise physiologists no longer use the slow- and fast-twitch classifications, preferring to call these fibers Type I (oxidative), Type IIa and IIab (oxidative and oxidative/glycolitic), and Type IIb (glycolitic), based on their need or lack of need for oxygen. We've chosen to use the older classification system because we think it's easier and clearer for the layperson.

though the ratios (which are set at birth) vary from muscle to muscle and person to person. Most great athletes, for instance, are genetically endowed with an abundance of big, fast fibers that give them the ability to explode off the line of scrimmage, slam a 95-mile-an-hour serve past an opponent, slap a puck into the net, or leap impossibly high to bring down a sure homer. They're simply not like the normal Joe, a fact that you can readily verify on any Sunday afternoon in the fall. If you watch an NFL game, you'll see big, fat linemen with their bellies hanging out, who look like they should be in front of the tube with a beer watching the game instead of earning millions of dollars blocking other big, fat linemen. How can these guys look so totally out of shape and be so quick and powerful? Luck of the genetic draw—they've got a high percentage of big, fast fibers to call on.

Contrast the physiques of the NFL linemen with those you see in body-building magazines—with their big, ripped, glistening muscles, these body builders make the NFL linemen look like a joke. So, why don't these perfectly chiseled body builders (who often weigh as much as the linemen) play in the NFL? Because, in most cases, they can't; they have neither the speed nor the explosive power required to compete in that arena. While they have trained to make their rippling muscles larger and stronger, they've been endowed with far fewer fast-twitch fibers.

When you join the Slow Burn Fitness Revolution, you vastly improve all your muscle fibers; you'll strengthen the slow ones, the intermediate ones, and even the fast ones. You'll make them all bigger and more metabolically fit, but you won't alter their ratios. Like it or not, you can only work with the genetic endowment you've got, with the goal of making yourself the leanest, strongest, healthiest you possible. (We'll explore this topic in even greater detail in a later chapter.)

This is good news for many women, who might want the health benefits of strength training but fear turning into the bulked-up freaks that grimace from the covers of muscle magazines. Set those fears aside. Women—without assistance from body-building steroids and other "muscle-building chemicals"—simply do not bulk to gargantuan proportions no matter how much iron they pump. They'll build some lean muscle, lose some fat, and become stronger, quicker, and more flexible. They'll build stronger bones and become more metabolically fit from their Slow Burn workout, but they won't turn into Ms. Incredible Hulk.

No matter what your gender is or what genetic hand you've been dealt regarding your muscle fiber makeup, age takes its toll. As we age, we watch our nimbleness and quickness fade, because our fast-twitch fibers begin to lose their strength and size. Things that once seemed easy—drifting over to snag a fly ball in center field, negotiating a mogul run on skis, bobbing and weaving through traffic for an easy layup, smashing a cross-court shot—become a challenge. As age continues to have its way with us, simpler things—putting cans of food on the shelf, lifting a small suitcase into the trunk or airline overhead bin, even carrying a bag of groceries—can exceed our capacity. The elderly can no longer do the simple things they took for granted in youth because time has robbed them of their muscle mass and, especially, the strength of their big, fast fibers.

Traditional weight workouts, particularly those designed for women and the elderly, usually involve sets of multiple repetitions using light weights ostensibly designed to reduce the risk of injury and increase stamina—or so the thinking goes. Unfortunately, it doesn't work that way. When you call upon a muscle to lift a given weight, the small, slow-twitch fibers respond first. If the weight is light, they can "tote the note" for many repetitions without fatigue. With more weight, however, these smaller fibers begin to fail, and the intermediate ones step up to the plate; they, too, can hang in for many repetitions with a lighter weight, lifted quickly. Only when the weight is heavy enough to fatigue both these fiber types do the fast-twitch fibers come off the bench and join the workout. And until they do, your workout isn't improving their size, their strength, or their metabolic health. Nor will it improve to any great degree your performance of activities that require bursts of power, whether that's smashing a forehand volley, cracking a line drive, lifting a toddler to your shoulders, or jumping out of the path of a bus. If you want to improve your performance in sports that require quick, explosive, powerful movements, such as tennis, football, baseball, racquetball, basketball, or skiing, or if you'd just like the simple strength-dependent activities of life to be simple again, you'll need to strengthen your big, fast-twitch fibers—however many you may have—and there's no quicker or more effective way to do that than by joining the Slow Burn Fitness Revolution.

The Slow Burn Technique

The revolutionary Slow Burn technique is designed to quickly bring about deep fatigue of the lesser muscle fibers and ignite a burn sufficient to fatigue even those powerhouses, the big, fast fibers. The key element is that each exercise must be performed with slow, precise repetitions, in perfect form, with a weight heavy enough to take the muscle being worked to total fatigue in just a few repetitions. Total fatigue is the point at which the muscle cannot move the weight anymore with any amount of coaxing. At that point, the muscle fibers send out a cascade of chemical signals that stimulate growth, increase strength, and improve metabolic functioning to ensure that should a similar work demand arise in the future, the muscle will be ready to meet the challenge. As a consequence, continued application of the technique quickly builds strength and restores the muscle mass, power, and quickness that have been lost to disuse or to age.

In a typical Slow Burn workout of a specific muscle group, you'll spend a mere sixty to ninety seconds perfectly performing a single set of only three to six repetitions. With each repetition, you'll take three seconds just to initiate the motion, allowing the muscle fibers to sit up and take notice that there's work to be done, then lift and lower the weight precisely and slowly. When performing a Slow Burn exercise with weights (either at home or in the gym), you'll want to select a weight so heavy that for the first second or two you feel like you won't be able to budge it. Just keep breathing calmly and pushing slowly, steadily, and with focus. If it's really too heavy, it won't budge. If you can lift the weight slowly, with good form, for at least sixty seconds, it is not too heavy. If you reach failure before about forty seconds, it's too much weight. If you can continue slow repetitions in perfect, slow form for longer than ninety seconds, the weight is too light. The ideal weight choice for any given exercise is one that allows you to complete three to six slow repetitions within the sixty-to-ninety-second time frame, before failure occurs. Your goal is to bring the muscle to utter fatigue—without letting momentum or gravity do any of the work for you—in good, slow form, not to lift a particular amount of weight.

Despite its terminal sound, "failure" isn't some catastrophic event during which the muscle collapses, but merely the point of deep, total fatigue at which no matter how hard you try you can no longer lift the weight and still maintain perfect, relaxed form. No twisting or arching your back, assisting with other body parts, grimacing, jerking the weight, or letting it fall with gravity. These maneuvers, so commonly seen in traditional gym settings, only invite injury and rob you of part of the benefit you would otherwise derive from your workout. Welcome failure—it is your sign of success and the targeted endpoint for each exercise.

If you spend a couple of minutes on each exercise with a minutes or so in between as you shift from one exercise to the next, you'll be able to complete the entire Slow Burn fitness regimen in less than half an hour and without breaking much of a sweat. You will have taken all your major muscle groups to deep fatigue, and in doing so, you'll have stimulated the growth and strengthening of all the muscle fiber types—including the big fast-twitchers—as you could do in no other way. And at the same time, you'll have reduced your risk of osteoporosis, increased your flexibility, improved your cardiovascular health, and, as you'll see in the next chapter, traded some body fat for muscle. Not bad for thirty sweat-free minutes a week.

Turn Your Body into a Fat-Burning Machine

I'm fat but I'm thin inside.

—GEORGE ORWELL

It's no secret that most Americans—indeed, most people in the westernized world—carry too much weight, or more correctly, too much fat. The majority of us could stand to shed a few pounds—a pair of love handles, a spare tire—but many of us need to lose substantially more. The truth is that most people who are overweight don't like it and would like to do something about it, if not for health reasons (of which there are many), then for reasons of self-esteem and aesthetics; unfortunately, however, they often find themselves confused on just how to go about it, and with good cause. Confusion reigns on the magazine shelves and talk-show circuit. Should you diet? Should you exercise? Which is better? The answer is that ideally, you should do both; proper diet sets the stage for maximal fat burning, and the right kind of exercise maximizes the loss.

Based on our nearly twenty years' experience helping overweight people lose weight effectively, we can tell you with absolute certainty that no exercise on earth—even Slow Burn—can make you lose excess body fat faster than simply eating a proper diet. To our minds, of course, "proper" means a diet rich in meat, fish, fowl, eggs, and dairy (all sources of high-quality protein), healthy fats, fresh fruits, and low-starch vegetables, and restricted in sugars, starches, and processed foods. It's a strategy that has helped millions of people, in America and around the world, lose weight and reclaim their health. We've provided some general nutritional guidelines and a full week of meal plans in Appendix C (page 173). If you'd like more details about this very effective nutritional strategy, you can find the full dietary program in *The Protein Power LifePlan* or in *Protein Power*, including which foods to eat, which ones to avoid, and why, along with meal plans and full instructions. But that said, when you're looking to maximize your fat loss—to really turn your body into a fat-burning machine so that you can reach your weight loss and health goals in the shortest time possible—there's no type of exercise that will aid your fat-loss effort more and get you to your goals faster than the Slow Burn Fitness Revolution. Why?

First, slow-motion strength training builds muscle better than any other form of training. In fact, studies show that slow-speed weight workouts build muscle about twice as fast as traditional weight training and faster by a mile than aerobics, jogging, walking, biking, or similar types of exercise. And the more muscle you build, the more calories your body will use in day-to-day living; the more calories you use, the faster you'll deplete your excess body fat. Second, Slow Burn training increases your body's sensitivity to the hormone insulin, the chief culprit behind weight gain. Elevated insulin levels signal the body to store excess incoming calories as fat and to prevent the breakdown of body fat for fuel—in effect, preserving your spare tire at all costs. As your body becomes more sensitive to insulin, your blood insulin level falls and, along with it, your blood pressure, cholesterol, and triglycerides. And, more significantly for weight loss, as insulin falls, the signal to pack calories away and hold them in the fat stores subsides, and it becomes much easier for you to lose body fat.

By combining proper diet with a thirty-minute-a-week Slow Burn workout, you'll set the stage for maximal loss of excess fat and be well on your way to the dramatic drops in belt and clothing sizes you've always hoped for but have never gotten. And best of all, continuing your Slow Burn workout will help to prevent the dreaded weight *regain* that plagues most people who lose weight following the standard diet and exercise prescription you may have tried before.

Does this story sound familiar? An overweight person finally decides to consult a doctor or dietician about losing weight; he or she comes away with a prescription to "eat less and exercise more." Restrict calories—especially calories from fat—and start walking or doing aerobics; that's the sure cure for excess weight. Or so conventional wisdom would decree. But is it? Can you simply "eat less and exercise more" and get the lean, healthy body you've dreamed of? Not really, and here's why.

When you eat fewer calories than you require to meet your body's energy needs, your body turns to its fuel stores—body fat and stored sugar—to make up the difference, by breaking down or burning up its tissues. If your body burns only excess body fat to meet its needs, that's perfect; unfortunately, that's not always the case. If in following the "eat less" prescription, you subsist on salads with fat-free dressings, diet drinks, and fat-free bagels with a smidgen of fat-free cream cheese, your body will recognize that it doesn't have nearly enough protein coming in for the day-to-day growth and repair of body tissues. To make up the difference, in addition to burning fat and stored sugar (glycogen) for energy, the body will begin to break down muscle that it will turn into the protein raw materials it needs for critical functions. Since muscle has weight, breaking it down and using it up results in weight loss on the scale—but not the kind of loss you're after. Studies have repeatedly shown that on a low-calorie (and usually protein-deficient) diet, as much as 30 to 40 percent of the weight lost is from muscle, bone, and vital organs. You don't want to lose muscle and vital tissues; you only want to lose excess fat, but sadly, by following the vague prescription to "eat less and exercise more," you may lose both. If you add aerobics to the mix, believe it or not, you can actually lose more muscle on a typical low-calorie eating plan than if you didn't exercise at all—a finding that's been published in a number of scientific research papers (and about which we'll have more to say later).

At first glance, it would seem impossible to lose muscle on the "eat less and exercise more" regimen because doing aerobics clearly seems to get you into better shape, and with the "eating less" part of the prescription, you can certainly lose some body fat. But the studies don't lie—too little food plus aerobic exercise often equals muscle loss. If you persevere with this prescription, you may end up at your ideal weight, perhaps even the weight you were at your high school graduation, but you won't end up looking like you did in high school; you'll have a very different body composition. Same weight, maybe, but with a lot more fat and a lot less muscle. Following the standard prescription for weight loss, if you're male, you'll typically go from being a big "apple" to being a smaller apple; if you're a woman, you'll shrink from a big "pear" to a little pear. Probably not the result you had in mind.

Then, to add insult to injury, once you've come to the end of your ride on the "eat less–exercise more" merry-go-round and you try to maintain your weight loss, you are more than likely doomed to failure, because your reduced muscle mass now burns so many fewer calories that unless you're prepared to stay on starvation rations forever, your weight inexorably creeps back up. Only this time, when you return to your original starting weight, you'll be worse off than you were before, because now you have less muscle (from eating less and exercising more, as well as from the loss that occurs with the march of time) and even more body fat. If you decide to take yet another crack at losing weight using the same old prescription, you'll fall into the futile cycle that we all know as yo-yo dieting. You need to break free of that cycle and try something different: join the Slow Burn Fitness Revolution! In contrast to aerobic exercise, which under certain circumstances can cause you to lose more muscle than if you did nothing, with a Slow Burn workout, you'll actually gain muscle as you lose fat.

Slow Burn turns your body into a fat-burning machine, not because of the extra calories you expend in the workout, but rather because of the metabolic and hormonal changes it brings about. Although the biochemistry of how this happens is quite complex, three basic forces are at work sending signals to turn on the fat-burning process, increase the number of fat-burning "furnaces" within the muscle cells, and preserve muscle mass. Let's take a moment to briefly explore how this works.

When you work a muscle to the point of failure, as you do with Slow Burn, it sends out hormonal signals to the rest of your body telling it to preserve the muscle at all costs. It's as if the body interprets the intense demand placed on the muscle as a verification of its worth: "We need this muscle for survival. Don't let anything happen to it. Move it to the head of the line. Give it the nutrients and fuel it needs to do this demanding and important job!" Once the body receives these signals, it will pretty much leave the muscle intact and go after your stored body fat—of which it can usually find plenty padding the butt and belly—to make up its caloric deficit.

Intense exercise—such as taking your muscle groups to failure with Slow Burn—also stimulates the production and activity of an enzyme (called AMP kinase) that appears to be the body's master fuel switch. Flipping that switch turns on the fat-burning process during exercise and keeps it going for a substantial amount of time after you quit. Studies have shown that the enzyme-stimulation switch stays flipped for about seven to ten days after a bout of high-intensity training—thus the need to perform a Slow Burn workout only once a week. That's why you'll continue to burn fat for days during the interval between workouts.

And finally, studies have also shown that high-intensity exercise such as Slow Burn causes as much as a fivefold increase in the number of "fat-burning furnaces" (called mitochondria) within the muscle cells. The more furnaces available per muscle cell, the more fat you can burn during your workout. The more muscle you build, the more furnaces you'll need to fuel them; the more furnaces you create, the more fat you'll burn. Get the picture?

Performing a regular thirty-minute Slow Burn workout once a week, then, builds and preserves muscle that prefers to burn fat as its fuel source, throws the switch to turn on the fat-burning process and keeps it on, brings more fat-burning furnaces online to meet the higher demand, and creates, in the process, an efficient fat-burning machine—you!

The Heart
of the Matter

CHAPTER 4

You should change your focus on exercise as
you age—you need to save those joints . . .
concentrate more on building muscle and less
on aerobics. —KENNETH COOPER, M.D.

(father of aerobics)

Stand on a downtown street corner and ask the first hundred people who walk by what a person has to do to build endurance. Odds are that all one hundred of them will say that you have to do some kind of "aerobic" exercise to develop endurance. Ask these same hundred people what *aerobic* means, and they will tell you it means jogging, biking, swimming, or doing "aerobics." If you then ask what aerobic exercise does for people, your subjects will tell you that it increases endurance because it strengthens the heart and lungs. If you were to tell them that aerobics doesn't really strengthen the heart and lungs—that instead it makes their muscles a little stronger and it just *seems* like their hearts and lungs work better—and if you were to then tell them that thirty minutes a week doing a Slow Burn workout will give them as much endurance as three hours of jogging, they would probably treat you like the village idiot and quickly move away.

Strange though it seems, your unlikely claim would be true. The Slow Burn strength-training regimen will give you greater general cardiopulmonary fitness and endurance than running.[1] The endurance you get from slogging along for miles every week comes not from any cardiovascular conditioning but from the strength that such a routine ultimately develops, as well as the sport-specific training effect that occurs. The heart and lungs don't get much stronger, if at all. The muscles in general, and in the legs and hips in particular, become stronger, and this increased *muscular* strength brings about the changes we call "getting in shape."

For example, if we were to remove Lance Armstrong's heart and lungs and place them into the body of a typical couch potato, this piece of surgical wizardry would not, in any way, allow that couch potato to win the Tour de France. In fact, it would not make the couch potato any healthier per se, unless he had heart disease and Lance didn't, which as you've learned already may or may not be present, even in the most amazing athletes.

George Sheehan, M.D., physician, writer, and running guru, pointed this out to his devotees years ago.[2] He wrote, "You might suspect from the emphasis on cardiopulmonary fitness that the major effect of training is on the heart and lungs. Guess again. Exercise does nothing for the lungs; that has been amply proved . . . Nor does it especially benefit your heart. Running, no matter what you've been told, primarily trains and conditions the muscles."[3]

[1]We use the phrase "general cardiopulmonary fitness and endurance" to contrast it with sport-specific endurance. Clearly, running will give you greater endurance for running, but not for such upper-body exercise as rowing, tennis, or racquetball, whereas the total-body strength gains from Slow Burn will enhance your endurance in almost any athletic pursuit.

[2]Like runner Jim Fixx, Dr. Sheehan was a fitness buff who advocated jogging and marathons for improved health but died decades short of the four score and eleven years allotted to the obese, inactive Winston Churchill.

[3]G. A. Sheehan, "Take the Muscles and Run," *The Physician and Sportsmedicine* 9 (1981): 35.

He's right. Running and other forms of "aerobic" exercise strengthen the muscles. Stronger muscles working more efficiently to draw oxygen from the blood reduce the demand on the heart and lungs, which gives the impression of improved cardiovascular or cardiopulmonary fitness.

You have the heart and lungs you're born with. Nature has designed them to last a good long while, and, assuming they're not diseased, they function pretty well right up to the end. Each of these organs has a limited performance capacity, and as long as you're working within that capacity, they seem to work just fine. When you exceed that capacity, however, the perception is that your heart and/or lungs are out of shape. As you age and lose muscle mass, activities you used to do with ease when you were stronger now become difficult; you pant and puff and your heart pounds when you try to do them. But that isn't because your heart and lungs have gotten weaker—your muscles have, and as a result, their inefficiency makes you exceed the comfort level and capacity of your cardiopulmonary system. You don't need to strengthen your heart and lungs; in fact, you can't. You need to strengthen your muscles so that they can once again function easily within the capacity of your heart and lungs.

The fact that increasing muscular strength can tremendously improve the "aerobic" condition of the heart and lungs is probably the most difficult thing to truly come to grips with because it seems so counterintuitive. Let's look at a common situation to better explain the concept before we get into what actually happens at the cellular level.

A man lives in a three-story walk-up apartment building. As he gets older, he notices that climbing the stairs daily becomes more and more of a chore. He is now almost sixty, and over the past few months he has really had to struggle. He begins to stop halfway up to rest and let his breathing and heartbeat slow down a little before climbing on. One day as he starts his climb, he hears his phone ringing, and without thinking he hustles up the stairs to get it. When he pushes open the door he is dizzy, his heart is pounding, and he is gasping for air. He staggers to the couch and drops. He lies there trying to catch his breath, the phone forgotten, as he begins to feel a tightening in his chest. As soon as his breathing slows enough for him to talk, he calls his doctor.

His doctor, being the cautious sort and fearing a heart attack in the making, tells his patient to immediately get to the emergency room, where, fortunately, everything checks out okay. His doctor, on a follow-up visit, tells the man that he needs to improve his cardiovascular fitness and encourages him to go to a cardiac rehab center, where he can start his "aerobic" regimen under the watchful eyes of the staff. Six weeks later, having spent three hours each week on a progressive cycling regimen, riding faster and faster against greater and greater resistance, he is released from the clinic and advised to continue his training program on his own at a gym.

He can now walk up the stairs without breaking a sweat. He reaches the top and he isn't even breathing hard. He hasn't felt this good in ten years. He is convinced that all of his diligent work has improved his heart and lungs. But has it?

Actually, no. He is stronger. His six weeks at the clinic strengthened his hips and legs. Now it is easier for him to walk up the stairs because he is stronger, just as he was years earlier when he zipped up the stairs without giving it a thought. His heart and lungs are pretty much the same; his redeveloped strength now allows him to work within their natural capacity.

But imagine how much more strength our subject would have developed had he spent just a fraction of those three hours per week doing Slow Burn training instead of mindlessly cycling away on a stationary bike.

Fine-Tuning the Muscle Machine

When you're sitting in front of the tube and the only exercise you're getting is popping another chip in your mouth and throwing back a swig of beer, your muscles, believe it or not, are mainly running on fat. That's right, fat. During times of little or no muscular activity, muscles primarily burn fat for their fuel. Muscle cells burn this fat in little sausage-shaped furnaces called mitochondria. Just like the furnace in your house, the mitochondria require plenty of oxygen to burn the fat, which is no problem if you're resting because the blood delivers all the oxygen they need and then some. If you jump up off the couch and head outside to shoot a little hoop, the situation changes; you start to burn a little glucose (blood sugar) along with your fat. As you increase the intensity of your activity, you begin to burn more and more glucose and less and less fat. When you're going all out, working or playing as hard as you can, your muscles are burning glucose and nothing else. But wait; don't you want to burn fat to lose weight and get fitter? While it may not seem like a good thing to stop burning fat, it actually is. Recall from earlier discussions that muscle fibers are recruited in increasing order of size and speed—the smaller, slower ones first and the biggest, fastest ones last. The small fibers burn mainly fat or a combination of fat and glucose. The big, explosively fast fibers burn purely glucose, so that when you finally call them into action, it's glucose you're burning, but in the process of getting to that point your muscles burned fat and will continue to do so for a prolonged period thereafter.

When you first start a fitness regimen and you are "out of shape" you wear out quickly; you end up puffing and panting with your heart pounding in fairly short order. After you've trained for a while you find that it takes a lot more activity to get your heart racing and your lungs burning. You reach a point at which the level of activity that originally wore you out doesn't even make you break a sweat. You're conditioned. To all appearances your heart and your lungs are in much better shape because now your heart doesn't beat as fast and your lungs don't have to suck in the air in gasps like they did before. But, appearances aside, are these organs functioning better? Or is something else going on?

Something else is going on. With a progressive exercise regimen heart function improves minimally, but lung function doesn't improve at all. Most of the improvement in heart function comes from what is called increased stroke volume, which means that the heart pumps out a little more blood with each beat. Although every little bit helps, the increase in stroke volume is just a drop in the bucket in terms of the overall changes that take place during the conditioning process.

The primary changes that take place, the ones that make all the difference, are metabolic. Metabolism can be loosely defined as all the actions and reactions that take place in the body to convert fuels to energy and to build up or break down tissues. Each of these metabolic functions, of which there are many, requires one or more enzymes to shepherd it along. Enzymes are the worker bees that produce all the chemical reactions necessary for our survival. Were it not for enzymes, we would all just be piles of chemicals sitting around taking years (or in some cases, centuries) to react. With the help of enzymes, however, these chemical reactions take place in fractions of seconds. As we'll see, Slow Burn, better than any other sort of exercise, maximizes the efficiency of metabolic functions.

The Law of Supply and Demand

Our bodies make enzymes as we need them, and the more we need, the more they make, but it's not an immediate process. A classic example is the enzyme that breaks down alcohol in the liver, alcohol dehydrogenase. When we take our first drink of alcohol, we have very little alcohol dehydrogenase in our livers, and it doesn't take very much alcohol to make us inebriated. If we continue to have a drink now and then, our bodies produce more alcohol dehydrogenase by a process called upregulation, and we can consume more alcohol without effect than we could when we took our first drink. Metabolic enzymes work in precisely the same way: we have to demonstrate a need for them, and ultimately the body will come through and provide them.

In order for a muscle to work it needs fuel (fat, glucose, or both) and oxygen. The fuels and oxygen must get into the muscle cells and then into the mitochondria. The metabolic systems that accomplish these fuel and oxygen transporting tasks are all driven by various enzymes, most of which the body is able to upregulate if needed. It is beyond the scope of this book to delve into all the scientific details of these complex metabolic systems, but we can present an overview of what happens when a muscle works and what happens when it is strengthened.

The enzymes that transport fat into the cell and then into the mitochondria are sort of loafing along when the muscle is at rest. The blood, coursing through the capillary network interwoven throughout the muscle, supplies plenty of oxygen to combine with the fat as it is oxidized (the scientific term for burning a fuel in the presence of oxygen) in the mitochondria. The energy released as the fat oxidizes is more than enough to meet the needs of the resting muscle. When the muscle begins to work, the fat-transport enzymes ratchet up their activity levels to move more fat into the mitochondria, a situation calling for more oxygen from the blood. If the muscle continues to work within its comfort threshold, all the processes hum along smoothly. As the muscle begins to work harder, however, things change.

As the muscle increases its activity, the fuel mixture changes from predominantly fat to a mixture of glucose and fat. And the working muscle requires more oxygen to keep up with the additional fuel requiring oxidation. If the muscle works even harder, the requirements for fuel and oxygen accelerate. The enzymes in an untrained muscle can do only so much, and at the point at which these enzymes are all working their hardest, the process of oxidation levels off. At this point the heart and lungs are doing their part to help: the heart is racing, pumping as much blood as it can to the working muscle; the lungs are filling the blood with as much oxygen as they can by drawing in huge gasps of air at a rapid rate. Despite all this effort on several fronts, the muscle would falter if it had nowhere else to turn for energy. But it does.

When the maximum amount of oxygen is being transferred and the muscle needs yet more energy, it turns as a last resort to the metabolism of pure glucose. In this process, called glycolysis, the body converts glucose to energy anaerobically (without oxygen). Anaerobic metabolism allows the muscle to keep working beyond the limit that would otherwise be quickly reached if it had to rely only on the oxygen-rich blood provided by the heart and lungs. The big, fast-twitch muscle fibers are the ones best equipped to use glucose anaerobically; the smaller, slow-twitch fibers burn fat and glucose aerobically, or in the presence of oxygen only.

In order for the muscle to use glucose anaerobically, the glucose must get into the muscle cells in large amounts quickly, which it does, driven by glucose transporters that are operated by enzymes. As the body converts glucose to energy to meet the muscle's needs, a byproduct is formed, called lactic acid. Lactic acid increases the acidity level of the blood around the working muscle and by a phenomenon known as the Bohr effect actually increases the amount of oxygen delivered to the muscle from the blood. The lactic acid travels from the muscle to the blood, then to the liver, where it is converted back into glucose, released into the blood, and transported back to the muscle for fuel. This glucose–lactic acid–glucose cycle is called the Cori cycle.

All these different systems, pathways, and cycles are enzyme driven. As you work out and gain muscle strength, these enzymes begin to work better and faster—that's the training effect. The muscle can work much harder before it reaches the point at which it runs out of steam because the enzymes that move the fuels and oxygen into first the cell and then the mitochondria work much more efficiently. And the number of mitochondria in the muscle increases dramatically, so there are many more furnaces to burn the fat and glucose. The amount of work you can perform without puffing and panting increases dramatically, not because your heart and lungs are working better but because all these enzymes systems are working better and are able to get all the oxygen they need from the blood even with a much slower heartbeat.

If you continue to push your muscles hard enough with a progressive strength-training program they will still revert to anaerobic metabolism when necessary, but only after a much longer period. And when they do revert to working anaerobically, they do that much more efficiently as well. The numbers of glucose transporters increase, ensuring the delivery of much more glucose into the cell; the enzymes of the Cori cycle all upregulate, providing a more rapid reconversion of lactic acid back to glucose. Glycolysis forms an intermediate byproduct called 2, 3-Bisphosphoglycerate (2, 3-BPG) that ultimately makes its way to the red blood cells, causing them to release oxygen to the working muscles more rapidly.

When you push your muscles to work anaerobically, you not only increase the activity of all glycolytic enzymes and pathways, you also help the aerobic pathways work better by providing more oxygen via the Bohr effect and the 2, 3-BPG effect. If you do only low-intensity training, such as jogging, walking, or cycling, only the aerobic enzymes are upregulated, and even then not to the extent they are when you force the muscle to work anaerobically. When you are working your muscles anaerobically as you do with a Slow Burn workout, both the aerobic system and the anaerobic system are operating at full tilt.

Another problem with low-intensity work is that instead of building your overall muscle mass, you can actually reduce it. If your muscles work aerobically, but just at the cusp of anaerobic, and they do it for a long time, say by running a marathon, they consume a large amount of glucose. The muscles do store some glucose, but when it is depleted, as it is in a long endurance event such as a marathon, the body has to get it somewhere. Unfortunately the body turns to muscle to get the additional glucose it needs; the muscle protein breaks down and is converted to glucose in a process called gluconeogenesis. You end up using the protein from the muscles not used for running to provide the glucose for the muscles that do need it. You can see why marathon runners have nicely developed legs and hips, but slight shoulders and arms—the so-called runner's physique. They typically also have haggard-looking faces, because the working muscles cannibalize the protein from the facial muscles as well, leaving the face without its base of support. The end result often turns out to be a loss of total lean body mass and a loss of overall muscle strength in exchange for improving cardiovascular fitness and endurance.

That doesn't have to be the case. Taking muscle groups to complete fatigue with a thirty-minute Slow Burn workout achieves an equally beneficial result. It delivers the dramatic improvement of the enzyme systems that is critical for what's generally thought of as cardiopulmonary fitness. But Slow Burn does it without the relentless jolting punishment of jogging, without the injury risks of roller-blading, and without the endless hours of time that these typical "get-in-shape" endeavors demand. When you understand the metabolic science behind getting fit, you realize that most of the ways we exercise are very roundabout and inefficient ways of building muscle strength. Why not do Slow Burn instead? In thirty minutes a week, you really can get right to the heart of the matter. What are you waiting for?

Enhancing Flexibility

CHAPTER 5

The human body ... indeed is like a ship; its
bones being the stiff standing-rigging, and the
sinews the small running ropes, that manage
all the motions.

—HERMAN MELVILLE (1819–91), *novelist*

Y ou wake up in the cool of the morning after a wonderful night's sleep and you stretch and twist, and it feels so good. You get out of the car after a three-hour trip and you stretch and twist your torso, and it feels great. You lean back in your chair after a session of hardwork on the computer and you stick your arms straight up, interlock your fingers, point your palms to the ceiling, stretching your weary wrists, and rock from side to side. And it feels terrific; you're relaxed, rejuvenated, and ready to compute some more. All these stretches and others like them bring pleasure that comes for the most part without risk of injury. But do they do us any good? It seems like stretching would make us more flexible, but does it? And what about regimented stretching programs such as yoga and Pilates? Do they do us any good? Do they improve our flexibility?

To answer these questions, we need to define our terms. What is flexibility? Flexibility is the ability to move a joint through its entire range of motion. A particular joint's range of motion depends upon a number of conditions: the integrity of the joint surface, the tightness and strength of the ligaments, the strength of the tendons, and the suppleness and strength of the muscles attached to the tendons. In fact, other than damage to the tendons and ligaments or to the joint surface itself, the most important factor in the kind of flexibility we want is muscular strength. Let's see why.

A joint is a connection between two different bones that allows them to move relative to one another and create mechanical force. Consider the hip joint, for example, a typical ball-and-socket joint. In this case the ball of the femur, the long upper bone of the thigh, moves relative to the pelvic bone, which contains the socket. The femur cannot only move back and forth, like a number of other joints, but it can rotate as well, giving you the ability to move your leg forward, backward, to the side, and across the other leg. The structure and mobility of the hip joints allow you to do the splits (or try), sit Indian style, squat, cross one knee over the other, and point your feet in and out. But you couldn't do any of these maneuvers if the "leg bone" weren't somehow attached to the "hip bone," as the old song goes. If there were nothing holding the ball in the socket, the muscles moving the leg relative to the hip would have nothing to act against.

Ligaments are the fibrous glue that holds joints together. In the case of the hip, a number of ligaments hold the ball tightly in the socket so that it can rotate in all directions but not come out of the socket. When a fall or other trauma exerts undue force on this joint, the ligaments can tear and release the ball from the socket, usually an extremely painful injury called a dislocation requiring forceful manipulation to get the ball back in the socket and a period of rest and immobilization to allow the ligaments to heal so they can once again hold the joint together. As you might imagine, ligaments that are loose will allow the joint more wiggle room and predispose it to dislocation. Loose ligaments will also allow the joint more freedom to move and increase flexibility, but at the price of a less stable joint—in most instances, not the best trade-off for greater range of motion and certainly not the best deal in the long run.

What determines the tightness of the ligaments? As with just about everything else concerning our bodies, it's genetics, to a great extent. The street performers you see who are hyperflexible, who can bend over backwards, stick their heads out between their legs, and do other seemingly impossible feats are born that way. You could practice for the next twenty years and never achieve that kind of flexibility, nor would you want to. Your ligaments would stretch, your joints would become loose, and you would be prone to dislocations in a way we will describe a little later.

While the ligaments hold the joints snugly in place, the muscles, acting through the tendons, actually move the bones. The tendons cross the joints and behave something like pulleys, allowing the bones to move relative to one another. In the case of the hip, the muscles of the upper leg are connected at one end by tendons attached to the leg and at the other end by tendons attached to the pelvis. As the muscle contracts it pulls the movable upper leg through a particular range of motion relative to the pelvis. Looking at another muscle/joint combination—the biceps and elbow—we can see this clearly. The biceps is connected to the lower arm via the tendon on one end and the upper arm by the tendon on the other. When the biceps contracts it pulls the lower arm toward the upper with the rotation of the two bones taking place through the joint (the elbow).

In addition to the actual joint surfaces, the ligaments that hold them in place, and the tendons that transmit the force that moves them, there is one more component of every joint—the muscles attached to the tendons. For example, if the biceps muscle can't contract (or can't lengthen), there will be very little active movement at the elbow. If you were to get a shot in your biceps that completely paralyzed it, your arm would hang straight down at the elbow; conversely, if you got a shot that intensely contracted your biceps, your hand would be stuck up by your shoulder, unable to be lowered. If either of these events took place, you could reasonably say that your elbow joint wasn't very flexible because it couldn't move through its normal range of motion. Despite the fact that your ligaments were working properly and your tendons were doing their job, your joint wouldn't move properly due solely to the action (or lack thereof) of your muscle. In this hypothetical example, the muscles are either artificially hypercontracted or relaxed, causing the joint to have little or no range of motion. In reality, however, just as in this exaggerated situation, the flexibility of all of our joints is largely determined by the strength and health of our muscles.

Stronger Muscles Make More Flexible Joints

We've all heard the warnings from coaches and other fitness gurus: don't lift weights or you'll become "muscle bound" and lose your flexibility. As it turns out, all these warnings are so much hogwash. Muscle strength actually *enhances* flexibility. Why? Because trained muscle is not only stronger, it is more supple, has improved circulation, is better hydrated, and can exert much greater force across the joint. Strong muscles moving the joint through its full range of motion while maintaining the integrity of the ligaments produce optimal, stable flexibility.

Unfortunately most people (including, sadly, many coaches) believe that the best way to improve flexibility is to stretch the joint. If you go to almost any gym and observe, you'll see trainers having their clients stretch through all sorts of contortions. And you will see people without trainers stretching their own shoulders, backs, hips, hamstrings, and anything else that they can conceivably stretch in the mistaken belief that they are gaining better flexibility. What they are gaining, in fact, is loose, unstable joints.

If you stretch one of your joints to the point of pain and burning to increase flexibility, you are stretching the ligaments that give the joint its stability. If you stretch a joint often enough and use enough force you will ultimately find that you indeed can move that joint through a greater range of motion. But you have increased the joint's range of motion because you have stretched and lengthened the ligaments. Now, instead of the ligaments holding the joint snugly in place, their looseness permits it to move around, allowing the increased range of motion, but also making the joint much less stable and much more prone to dislocation. Let's look at an example to see what happens to joints that have been stretched to the point of instability.

A thirty-five-year-old retired professional ballerina begins to suffer occasional mild dislocations of her shoulders while reaching over her head, or of her hips if she steps up on a stepstool or something else a little elevated. When this happens she experiences some minor discomfort, but she is able to manipulate her shoulders or hips until the joints relocate. As she ages these minor dislocations become more frequent, more painful, and more difficult to get back into place. She consults her physician who tells her to begin a progressive exercise program, starting out with—you guessed it—brisk walking.

She starts her regimen, and a few weeks later, while walking briskly, she makes a small leap over a mud puddle, tears a ligament in her hip joint (due to its looseness and resultant instability), and experiences a complete hip dislocation. She collapses from the excruciating pain. The fall fractures her hip, twists her knee, and also dislocates the unstable shoulder with which she tries to brace herself on the way down.

After a week in the hospital and thousands of dollars' worth of orthopedic surgery, she returns home to remain immobile for a month while everything heals. Then it's off to an extended course of physical therapy—more dollars spent, more time away from her job and family. And the joints not repaired by the surgeon are still unstable and waiting for just the wrong move to cause a replay of the whole expensive mess. Our ballerina is now a forty-year-old basket case whereas fifteen years before she was a remarkable physical specimen renowned for her incredible strength and flexibility. What happened?

She was able to perform at a professional level by virtue of the fact that she was genetically "gifted" with loose-ligamented joints, allowing her to flawlessly perform all the difficult and precise movements her profession demanded. Compensating for this joint instability was her strength, which came, to some extent, from the strengthening effects of her ballet training and endless hours of practice and, to a greater extent, from her youth. As she aged, she lost both muscle mass and strength until she, like—ultimately—all elite athletes, couldn't keep pace with the younger, stronger practitioners of her discipline. In due course, she took her final bows and hung up her toe shoes for the last time.

After her retirement her activity level declined precipitously, further accelerating her age-related loss of muscle mass and strength. With time and continued strength loss, her muscles became less and less able to overcome her joint laxity until she reached the point where our story began, when she was experiencing partial dislocations. If instead of letting age take its course, she had begun a regimen of Slow Burn strength training upon her retirement, she would have become stronger than she had ever been before in fairly short order. Her increased strength would have more than compensated for her dislocation-prone joints, allowing her to lead a normal, injury-free life. Had she begun strength training before her retirement, she more than likely could even have extended her career.

What lessons does the story of our ballerina's travails hold for the rest of us who never plan to be professional dancers? Simply this. Don't allow a regimen of serious stretching to do to you what genetics did to the ballerina. Instead, maximize the flexibility you do have with Slow Burn strength training.

The medical evidence shows that all the components of the joint improve with strength training. Scientists have compared the strength of both ligaments and tendons before and after strength training and have found that these structures uniformly become stronger, allowing more motion of the joint without the danger of dislocations, sprains, or tendon ruptures. This increased ligament and tendon strength, coupled with the tremendous increase in muscular strength and elasticity resulting from Slow Burn training, gives joints enhanced flexibility as well as a dramatically decreased risk of injury. A stretching regimen, on the other hand, does just the opposite—it increases joint flexibility at the price of increased risk of dislocation.

What about other types of training? Do other activities besides strength training strengthen the joints and provide more (and safer) flexibility? Not really, and not very much. Any activity that increases strength is going to increase flexibility, but, as we've seen, nothing increases strength as quickly as Slow Burn training, so, by extension, nothing will increase flexibility as quickly either.

Recently researchers at Democritus University of Thrace in Greece, the birthplace of the Olympics, had some of these same questions. They initiated a study comparing the flexibility subjects gained with strength training, aerobic training, and a combination of the two. The researchers recruited a number of elderly, sedentary men (average age about 70) and divided them into four randomized groups: a group of controls, who did nothing; a group that undertook an intensive strength-training program of weight lifting only; a group that engaged in vigorous aerobics only (jogging and walking at 50 to 80 percent of maximum heart rate); and a group that did both strength training and aerobics. All subjects were evaluated for seven different measures of flexibility of their knees, hips, shoulders, elbows, and lower backs before, during, and after sixteen weeks of training. At the beginning of the study the men in all four groups had the same degree of flexibility (or inflexibility).

At completion of the training period, the strength-trained subjects had enormous increases in flexibility in all seven categories. The men who jogged and walked did show minimal increases in flexibility, but only in their hips, and their improvement was nothing compared to that achieved by their strength-trained counterparts. Moreover, they showed no increases in flexibility in any of the other areas measured. These men could have sat on their duffs like the sedentary group instead of running almost three hours a week and, apart from minimal increases in hip flexibility, experienced the same changes as the control group, i.e., none. The group of men who did both strength training and aerobic training increased their flexibility to the same degree as those who underwent strength training alone.[1] Clearly, if it's improvement in flexibility you want, strength training is the way to get it.

In their textbook on athletic training, *Scientific Basis of Athletic Conditioning*, Brigham Young University professors and exercise physiologists Clayne Jensen and Garth Fisher report that among athletes, Olympic weight lifters were second only to gymnasts in their overall score on a number of flexibility tests. Think of it. You have boxers, figure skaters, pole vaulters, high jumpers, javelin throwers, swimmers, and athletes from all the other competitive categories in the Olympics, and none except for the gymnasts are as flexible as the weight lifters. How did these weight lifters get to be so flexible? Was it yoga? Pilates? A regimen of painful stretching exercises? No. Their secret is that they have great muscular strength and, accordingly, strong ligaments and tendons, allowing the joints to move easily through their entire range of motion.

Do you want to enhance your flexibility? Forget about stretching, yoga, Pilates, and all the rest. Do Slow Burn for thirty minutes a week instead and make your joints be the best that they can be.

[1] I. M. Fatouris, et al. "The Effects of Strength Training, Cardiovascular Training and Their Combination on Flexibility of Inactive Older Adults." *International Journal of Sports Medicine* 23 (2002): 112–119.

Stronger Bones

CHAPTER 6

A bone is a living organism. Strength
training makes it stronger. Lack of
tension weakens it. — WERNER
KIESER, *founder, Kieser Training centers*

A silent epidemic is raging in America: weak bones. Currently, an estimated 26.2 million American women have some degree of bone loss and weakness. In nearly 17 million of these women, the disease has already caused detectable bone thinning, or osteopenia; in over 9 million more, it has progressed to the severe bone mineral loss we know as osteoporosis, a disease that will sharply raise their risk for sustaining serious fractures as they age. Although we often tend to think of osteoporosis as a disease peculiar to older women, it commonly affects men, as well; in fact, after age 50, osteopenia or osteoporosis will affect not only one in three women, but also one in twelve men. And every year, thanks largely to this epidemic of bone weakness, 1.5 million older Americans will break a bone: their backs, their forearms, or, more ominously, their hips. Some of them—especially frail elderly men, who for reasons that aren't clear don't fare well under the stresses of such hip injuries—will die of hip fracture complications. Are we to assume that as our population ages we must all trudge forward toward this fate? Not at all! Let's first take a brief look at bones. What causes them to weaken, and what can we do to make them strong?

Building Strong Bones

Ask just about anyone what kids need to build strong bones, and they're likely to tell you, "plenty of nutritious food, lots of milk for calcium, and plenty of time spent romping and playing in the sunshine." And they'd be absolutely right. From before birth through adolescence, kids are obviously growing bigger and taller, and their bones have to lengthen and strengthen to meet these demands. This isn't news. But what many people don't realize is that once children reach adulthood and this period of rapid lengthening and development stops, bone growth goes on. The focus shifts away from making bones longer and thicker to center on the upkeep, maintenance, and repair functions that keep them healthy and strong—at least until about age thirty, when, like most other organ systems in the body, bone mass begins to decline with age . . . that is, if we don't work to maintain it.

Based on the skeletons displayed in museums or hanging in a physician's office, you may be tempted to think of adult bones as rock-hard, lifeless sticks; nothing, however, could be further from the truth. Bones are vital, living tissues that constantly build, remodel, and renew. Bone is built of hard minerals laid down upon a living framework of fibrous protein fabric called collagen. As bone ages or wears, the body breaks down and absorbs the old or damaged areas of the framework and the mineral matrix that fills it and replaces them with strong new bone. Ideally, the removal and restoration processes remain in balance, and the bones stay healthy and in good repair. If removal exceeds replacement, however, weak bones result. What does it take to keep bones strong? Plenty of the nutritional raw materials to build them, and the right chemical and hormonal signals from within that stimulate growth and repair.

On the nutritional end, thanks to the dairy lobby and its milk-mustache campaign, just about everyone is familiar with the need for the most abundant mineral in bone, calcium; unfortunately, they're far less familiar with its equally important mineral partners magnesium and phosphorus, as well as boron and a host of other trace minerals. All of these minerals—along with adequate vitamin D from fish, eggs, liver, or exposure to sunlight—are important to bone health and should be a part of any bone-building regimen you undertake.[1] To build and maintain the collagen framework of bone, you'll also need an adequate daily amount of high-quality, complete protein, ideally from meat, eggs, fish, and dairy products.

Just as in childhood, bone health in adulthood depends upon an orchestrated interplay of genetics, good nutrition, growth factors and hormones (especially the reproductive hormones estrogen, progesterone, and testosterone), sunlight, and mechanical stress or use. That's right, *use*. Bones are made to bear weight, to do work. When they're stressed, they adapt, grow, and become strong; when they're not asked to do their load-bearing job, they quickly become thin, weak, and frail. Disuse is deadly to a healthy bone.

Numerous studies have shown that during prolonged periods of disuse—for instance, in patients on medically necessary bed rest or astronauts living or traveling in space without gravity—the bones markedly weaken and become thinner. Granted, these are extreme and unusual situations, but the same thing, in less dramatic fashion, happens day after day, year after year to otherwise healthy adults who

[1] For a more complete discussion of sunlight and supplementation for bone health, see Michael R. Eades, M.D., and Mary Dan Eades, M.D., *The Protein Power LifePlan* (New York: Warner Books, 2000).

adopt a sedentary lifestyle—and nowadays, that's a great many people.

On the other hand, active weight bearing builds and strengthens the bones. And therein you'll find the one and only health benefit of obesity: strong bones. Obese people put tremendous stress on the bones of their hips, legs, ankles, and feet just in the day-to-day activities of living. For instance, a 350-pound person rising from a chair is doing a pretty hefty leg press; in the same individual, climbing stairs amounts to a single leg press, effectively doubling the workload. Although obesity comes with too high a health cost otherwise to make it a useful way to prevent osteoporosis, it's easy to achieve the same benefit without the risks: simply join the Slow Burn Fitness Revolution.

Let's examine in a little detail a recent study published in the *International Journal of Sports Medicine* that points up the clear benefit—and safety—of strength training. While research has repeatedly shown the beneficial effect of strength training on building bone, concern has been voiced from some corners about the safety of weight lifting, particularly for the low back. Previous studies done on cadaver bones have determined a hypothetical maximum force that the average human lumbar vertebra (low back bone) can withstand before collapsing. Based on such studies, it's long been assumed that applying a force on the lumbar spine that exceeded this hypothetical maximum might result in collapse or fracture of the bones—not the outcome you'd want if bone building were your goal. To test this assumption, the research team undertook a study to examine the lumbar bone mineral density (a measure of bone mass and strength) of a single individual: the gentleman who happened to be the world record holder for the squat lift—his record was an incredible 469 kilograms, or nearly 1,100 pounds. X-ray studies determined that his low back was completely healthy, the alignment normal, with no evidence of compression, herniation, or disease of his disks, despite the incredible force applied to them by this amazing amount of weight. But it was the density scan of his lumbar spine that really astonished the researchers: his was the highest bone mineral density ever recorded. And this single case more than doubled the previous hypothetical maximum for safe compressive force of the low back.

Apart from this one intriguing study, however, dozens of other medical studies have demonstrated the clear benefits to bone health that accrue from strength training: increased bone density in the hips, lumbar spine, and arms—all sites of high fracture risk; dramatic gains in muscle strength; and substantial improvement in dynamic balance. Together, these benefits add up to fewer falls and fewer broken bones.

Sure, you can achieve some increase in bone density from doing other types of intense weight-bearing exercise, such as jogging or aerobics, but studies have shown that the gains in mineral density are less dramatic with these activities than with strength training and that they occur primarily in the low back, less in the hips, and hardly at all in the arms and shoulders. Then, of course, you have to factor in the added cost of what the repetitive trauma of jogging mile after mile does to the hip, knee, and ankle joints—not to mention the higher risk of injury from twisted ankles, shinsplints, skinned knees, dog bites, or being run down by an inattentive driver.

So, how about walking? Although walking is certainly a weight-bearing activity and clearly less traumatic to joints than jogging or aerobics, studies have failed to show that walking does much to preserve or build bone density, despite its sterling reputation as an easy-for-anyone-to-do exercise, its reputed health benefits, and the stress-relieving pleasure it brings to many people.

Interestingly, under certain circumstances some of these activities can prove counterproductive to building up your bone strength. For example, some studies have shown that if you couple jogging or aerobics with a very low-calorie diet— the very prescription many weight-conscious women at or near menopause follow—you might even cause further *weakening* and thinning of the bones of the low back and the femoral neck (the bone bridge that joins the ball of your hip to your upper leg, and a common location of serious hip fractures). Imagine all your hard work causing further bone loss instead of promoting a gain in strength and density— not at all the outcome you'd seek from your efforts.

No, the hands-down bone-building winner is weight lifting, but before you grab a set of light dumbbells and start cranking out the reps, take a look at this intriguing bit of research. A recent study compared two groups of women involved in exercise to strengthen their bones. One group lifted lighter weights with many repetitions, in what was termed an "endurance" protocol; the other group of women lifted heavier weights with fewer repetitions, in what was termed a "strength" regimen. What the researchers found, and probably surprisingly so, was significant bone mass increase with the strength regimen, especially in the all-important hip region, but *no increase whatsoever* with the endurance protocol. The researchers concluded that the peak load— that is, the heaviest weight that can be properly lifted—was more important than the number of repetitions.

Without reservation we can say that a properly performed regular total-body strength-training regimen such as the Slow Burn Fitness Revolution brings about bigger and better-sustained bone-density gains in men and women of all ages—even those in their eighties and nineties—than any other form of exercise. Whether for you such improvement translates into better athletic performance, less risk of osteoporosis later in life, rebuilding bones already weakened and thin, or better endurance in everything from recreational sports to climbing stairs to lifting your groceries or your grandkids, a once- or twice-a-week Slow Burn session is the key to healthier bones and better balance, with more time left over to enjoy doing things you once thought you couldn't do.

Bye-Bye, Back Pain

CHAPTER 7

Never grow a wishbone, daughter, where
your backbone ought to be.
—CLEMENTINE PADDLEFORD
(1898–1967), *food editor*
New York Herald Tribune

At some point in their lives, 80 percent of adults will fall victim to painful disorders of their low backs; it is the most common cause of disability for people before age forty-five, and second only to the common cold as a cause for a visit to the doctor. Each year, in the United States alone, the total costs related to back pain and injury top $50 billion. Back disorders account for nearly a third of the occupational injuries involved in lost work. Why is it so common for our backs to break down? The primary blame can be laid at the door of a widespread loss of muscle and soft tissue strength in the lumbar spine. To better understand how and why this occurs, let's take a look at how the back is put together.

Like all parts of the spinal column, the lower back, or lumbar spine, is at its core a relatively simple structure. It consists of a column of chunky bones (vertebrae) stacked one upon the other, with cushioning spacers (disks) between them in a design that provides a resilient, protective covering for the delicate spinal cord housed within. This basic simplicity, however, belies the complex network of small joints and soft tissues made of muscles, tendons, and ligaments that attaches the five lumbar vertebrae to each other, permitting movement and providing support to the basic structure.

On either side of each bone in the back, nerves exit the spinal column on their way to the various parts of the body, to which they provide the electrical stimulus for movement and sensation. Much of the pain and disability that occurs with lower back problems arises when weakness of or injury to the bones or soft tissues causes the basic spinal structure to collapse, resulting in pressure on the nerves.

The lower back also serves as the bridge that connects the torso (chest and arms) to the pelvis and legs and, in that role, provides the strength and mobility for such activities as twisting, turning, and bending. We must have a strong and stable lower back to walk, stand, sit, stoop, squat, or lift; in short, a healthy low back is critical for virtually every activity of normal daily living. And yet, as we pass the age of thirty, the lower back often becomes our weakest link. Why?

A variety of factors, such as genetics, age, disuse, and injury, can conspire to cause this common affliction. Unless we act to prevent it, the march of time robs us of muscle mass, bone mass, and strength in the low back, as elsewhere in the body. As the strength in the lumbar muscles ebbs, the force of gravity overwhelms the muscular support structure, and, as a result, the spaces between the vertebrae start to narrow. In addition, the slick cartilage covering the joints becomes roughened and stiff with age, the joints fall victim to the ravages of arthritic wear and tear, and the disks, ligaments, and tendons lose much of their resilience and natural elasticity. All of these factors weaken the back. Granted, accident and injury play a role, but far and away the most critical factor in the development of most low back pain is loss of muscle mass and strength. Although we can't stop the clock, we can regain the strength and stability of the muscles and soft tissues that support the low back by using them properly.

You'll recall from earlier discussions that both bone and muscle will quickly dwindle in size and strength if left to lie idle. Forced bed rest, immobilization of a limb in a splint or cast, and prolonged states of weightlessness (space travel, for instance) all inevitably result in significant losses of muscle mass, bone mass, and strength. Conversely, asking the muscles to do significant work—to lift a load, to repeatedly contract and relax across the joints to which they attach— results in the release of biochemical signals that stimulate growth, strengthening, and repair of the muscles and the supportive connecting tissues. Strength training would seem, then, a simple and obvious answer to lower back weakness and disability, and indeed, it is. Improving the strength of the lumbar muscles and connective soft tissues has long been recognized by orthopedists, chiropractors, and physical therapists as the cornerstone of low back rehabilitation. There is no question that regular strength training of the lumbar spine will both prevent and resolve low back pain. The challenge is how to accomplish this goal.

As you now understand, making significant gains in muscle strength and restoring losses in bone and muscle mass quickly means taking the target muscle to complete failure in perfect form. To do so properly, you must isolate the muscle or group of muscles in question and work them in such a way that momentum, gravity, and other parts of the body can't assist the effort. While this "isolation policy" is pretty easy to achieve with the shoulder muscles, biceps, or quads, for instance, it's much more difficult in the case of the lumbar muscles, because the much stronger muscles in the buttocks and the backs of the legs tend to get into the act and do the work. Consequently, it's almost impossible to get a proper lumbar workout at home or using free weights.

The lumbar muscles can only be effectively isolated using a lumbar extension machine. Lumbar extension machines are designed with a series of restraints that prevent tilting of the pelvis, rotation around the hip joints, or contribution from the big, strong muscles of the buttocks and thighs that would interfere with the work of the low back muscles. Even though it may prove to be something of a hassle, if you suffer from, have a family history of, or are occupationally at risk for low back problems, the effort you expend in locating and regularly using this piece of equipment will reward you with a healthy lumbar spine. (See Appendix A for help in finding a facility that sells or has such a device.)

A word of caution applies here: If you currently suffer from any serious low back disorder—particularly a disk problem—you should consult your physician or physical therapist before beginning Slow Burn or any strength-training regimen. That said, once you've got the green light from your health-care provider, there's no safer or more effective method for preventing or resolving this pervasive disorder.

The rules for igniting a Slow Burn in the lumbar muscles are exactly like those for any other muscle group (and are spelled out clearly on page 27): apply steady pressure against the load to move the weight about one inch per second in both the lifting and lowering phases of the exercise. With excruciating slowness, take three seconds to move the weight the first inch, at least seven seconds to lift, three to reverse directions, and seven to lower to the starting position. Don't jerk, twist, grimace, clench your teeth, or hold your breath.

Don't let momentum or gravity do part of your work. Continue to smoothly lift and lower the weight until you simply cannot move the weight again. Take the lumbar muscles to complete failure in three to six reps once a week and say, "Bye-bye, back pain!"

Improving Athletic Performance

CHAPTER 8

Exercise is the goddam key;

the more I do, the better I get.

—TED WILLIAMS (1918–2002)

Boston Red Sox Hall of Famer

The Genetics of Performance

As medical science advances, researchers are coming to understand more and more the enormous difference genetics makes in health and other areas of life. For instance, the celebrated runner Jim Fixx, whom you'll recall from Chapter 1, was a victim of his genetics; his father died at an early age from a heart attack, and despite his endurance and fitness, so did he. Winston Churchill obviously had much better longevity genes than Jim Fixx, living into his nineties despite a much more sedentary and hedonistic lifestyle. Fortunately, or unfortunately as the case may be, we are all endowed with our own unique genes. We can't change them; all we can do is make the best of them.

But our genetic makeup doesn't involve just our health and longevity; it also plays a large role in determining our basic physical appearance, our natural talents and abilities, and our response to training. To a great extent, our genetic makeup influences the level of athletic prowess we can achieve because it determines the relative amounts of the various fiber types in our muscles.

For example, a question on the minds of many women

who consider strength training is: Will I bulk up? They don't want to look like the women they see in bodybuilding magazines and are a little bit apprehensive that strength training will make them look more like men than women. Not to worry, it won't happen. The women in bodybuilding magazines are one in ten thousand in terms of their genetic ability to bulk up, and in most cases, the really grotesquely overdeveloped ones have had a little help from their friends, the anabolic steroids (testosterone and its chemical cousins). Studies have shown that pound for pound, muscles of any age group or gender are equally strong; female muscles are just as strong as those in men. If you are female, you will definitely become stronger as you strength train. Along with your increased strength, you'll be rewarded with a leaner, trimmer, but still feminine appearance. You'll develop attractive muscle definition that screams "strong and healthy!" but you won't risk developing massive bulk. The extra X chromosome that's part of your genetic makeup (and that determines that you are, indeed, female) will protect you from over-bulking as you train.

Unlike women, men who start strength training often *do* want to end up looking like the men they see in bodybuilding mags. But while men do have naturally higher levels of male hormones (such as testosterone) that make it relatively easier for them to build muscle, if they don't have the specific genetics for really bulking up, it won't happen. It doesn't matter how hard they work or, for that matter, how many anabolic steroids they take—they won't look like the guys in the magazines unless they've got the genes for it. Yes, they'll build nice, healthy, strong muscles. Yes, they'll look lean and fit. But most of them will not see their picture on the cover of *Muscle Media 2000*.

If nature has endowed you with muscle bellies that are

short and are connected to the joints with long tendons, you can work out until the cows come home and you will never look like Arnold. You can become strong as an ox, you can develop a superb physique, but you're never going to win a bodybuilding contest. If you want to get "ripped" and "shredded," you've got to have the genetics for it. If you do have the genetics for it, Slow Burn will "rip" and "shred" you faster than any other method around.

A book written around ten years ago by an aspiring bodybuilder about his experiences in the world of competitive bodybuilding highlights just how much of a role genetics plays.[1] The author was a skinny kid who, after returning from his education at Oxford, started working as an editor. He took up strength training and in short order found himself seduced into the hard-core bodybuilding subculture. He abandoned his job to devote himself full time to his new avocation, moved to "Muscle Beach," California, and got heavily into anabolic steroids and a host of other chemical muscle enhancers. Despite his full-time efforts, and despite multiple cycles of various anabolic steroid regimens and consumption of hundreds of grams of protein and a dozen supplements every day, he never managed to even get close to winning any kind of competition. His "before" picture shows a tall, slender young man; his picture in his bodybuilding prime shows a physique that anyone would be proud of but that would never grace the cover of a bodybuilding magazine. The point is that he didn't have the genetics, so despite his best efforts, he couldn't overcome the body nature gave him. Like all of us, he has to do the best he can with what he has.

The same holds true for athletic performance. As we'll see

---

[1]Samuel Wilson Fussell, *Muscle: Confessions of an Unlikely Bodybuilder* (New York: Avon Books, 1992).

later in this chapter, Slow Burn training will help you maximize the athletic ability you have, but it won't necessarily make you into a superstar. Three things determine your athletic ability: genetics, skill, and strength. You can improve your skill by practice and you can vastly improve your strength with Slow Burn, but you can't do anything about your genetics.

Dan Marino, the great quarterback for the Miami Dolphins, was notorious for avoiding the weight room. But his skill level and his genetics were enough to allow him to play at the highest level for many, many years and set countless NFL records. Could he have played better if he had done regular strength training? Undoubtedly. But his genetics made him so good that he could still perform at a superstar level without it. Could he have played longer? Probably. As he aged, Marino lost strength and muscle mass each year, as all of us do. He finally reached a point at which his incredible natural talent and skill could no longer sufficiently offset the inevitable loss of strength and endurance that comes with age; when his overall performance began to suffer, he hung up his helmet. That is the trajectory of every superstar's career, from Babe Ruth to Wayne Gretzky. The superstars who continue to strength train—Nolan Ryan comes immediately to mind—can extend their careers considerably and remain at the top of their game.

Barry Bonds, the San Francisco Giants slugger, has the genetics, the skill, and the strength to play in the major leagues and has had it for years. If you see pictures of him a few years back, you'll see a thin, rangy guy. He was a good player, but it wasn't until he began strength training that he became the powerhouse home run hitter that he is today. From his current picture, he's barely recognizable as the same player pictured years before—and his home run statistics have been transformed just as completely. Although there is a controversy raging today over whether or not Bonds used anabolic steroids to help himself develop strength and bulk, the fact remains that however he did it, he certainly increased the strength factor in his athletic equation, and in doing so catapulted himself into the record books.

A Rising Tide Lifts All Boats

How, you may be wondering, can doing a single type of exercise improve your performance in all others? How can doing Slow Burn make you a better batter or make it easier to blow a service ace by your opponent on the court, or add twenty or thirty yards to your drives on the links? Don't you have to cross-train or something?

The received sports wisdom has long been that to improve your performance in any activity you should practice that activity—only more so. For instance, batters standing in the on-deck circle add weights to their bats as they take practice cuts to warm up. The same technique has been applied variously to tennis racquets and golf clubs. In theory, when the weight is removed, the equipment should feel light as a feather and easier to whip around with more speed and power. However, when this theory is tested, it just doesn't pan out, because the specific muscle fibers called upon to swing the heavier bat aren't the same as the ones used for the lighter bat. In effect, it's a different activity. There is no doubt that muscles do entrain in response to repeated performance of an activity; it's called practice. But in point of fact, what practice builds is *skill* not *strength*. So if you want to improve your skill in hitting a baseball, you take regular batting practice with the same equipment you intend to use in actual play. If you want to improve your tennis serve or your backhand, or your strokes at the net, you get on the court and practice over and over and over to build your skill. Don't the hours of regular practice make you stronger? Yes, to a degree, but not as effectively as specifically working at that goal through strength training. And here's why.

As you'll recall from Chapter 2, activities that require explosive power, such as hitting a baseball, smashing a service ace, hitting a tee shot, or jumping out of the path of an oncoming bus, call upon the services of the big, fast-twitch muscle fibers; they're what totes the load in all such instances. Unfortunately, these same activities don't *build* the strength and mass of the big, fast fibers. Remember, to effectively build muscle and increase strength, you've got to take the muscle to complete fatigue, utterly exhaust it. And you can't do that with a few strong cuts of the bat followed by a long period of rest until the next time you're up. You can't bring these fibers to fatigue with one or two serves and periods of rest punctuated by single returns. Or with a single tee shot every fifteen minutes. You simply can't fatigue the big fibers with intermittent activity. It's paradoxical that the very activities that demand the explosive power of your big fast-twitch fibers won't improve them. But you can bring them to utter fatigue with a single Slow Burn workout each week. And by doing so, you'll make all your muscle fibers bigger and stronger and more capable of performing whatever explosive endeavor you ask of them—if you have the skill to perform it. Now that's cross-training!

Will following a Slow Burn regimen turn you into a Dan Marino or a Barry Bonds? A Tiger Woods or a Venus Williams? Not unless you have been born with their genetic gifts and have developed their level of skill. But will Slow Burn make your golf drives go farther? You bet. Will it make the ball fly off your tennis racquet at a blazingly faster speed? Absolutely. Will skiing be easier, faster, and less exhausting? Without a doubt. Will juggling bags of groceries while trying to deal with small children, strollers, and other paraphernalia be less trying? Yes! There is no activity or task or sport imaginable that won't be easier if you are stronger. And there is simply no better way to get stronger fast and without a major time commitment than with Slow Burn training. So as the swoosh people say: Just do it!

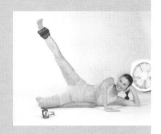

Part Two

THE *SLOW BURN* TOTAL-FITNESS ROUTINE

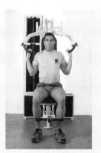

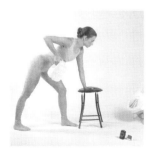

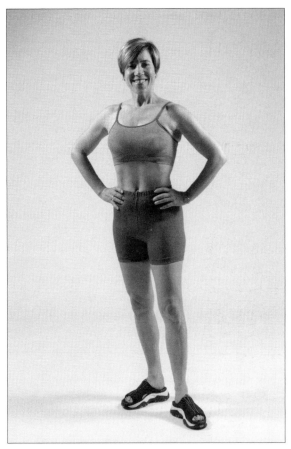

When I first heard about Fred Hahn's Serious Strength gym I thought, "C'mon, this can't be for real! Only thirty minutes a week and no aerobics?" I figured, well, what the heck and gave it a try. Lo and behold, I lost thirty pounds *and* four sizes *in just a few months. The combination of slow strength training and eating properly is really amazing. When I looked in the mirror, it was almost like I was looking at someone else. I recommend Slow Burn training* to everyone. *It's the most incredible thing I've ever done for my body!*

—KATHLEEN HAYS
FINANCIAL REPORTER, CNN

Overview

Now that you clearly understand how the Slow Burn Fitness Revolution works not only to make you stronger but to burn fat, restore your muscle and bone mass, enhance your flexibility, and improve your cardiovascular health as well, it's time to put its power into action and begin your journey toward becoming that stronger, leaner, healthier person you know you can be. The first and most critical step in this process is making the decision that you're ready to take charge of your fitness, reclaim your health, and strengthen your weak bones and muscles. Ask yourself now if you're mentally ready to change your life and reclaim your health. In the coming chapters, you'll learn exactly how to do it.

If you skipped over Part One and flipped right to this section to start your routine, be sure to go back and read at least the section on Slow Burn Technique on pages 27–29. It's crucial to your success that you clearly understand the overall method and the rationale for reaching success through failure.

Unlike most exercise regimens, which require you to commit hours to the activity several times each week—hours that you simply may not have available in a busy life—

joining the Slow Burn Revolution will cost you a mere half hour a week. In the time it would take to watch an episode of *Friends*, you can change your shape, double your strength, restore your bone and muscle mass, reclaim your health, and improve your life. If you're ready to go, all you have to do is decide where and how you want to train. Will it be in your own home or office or in a gym or fitness center? Would you prefer to train on your own, with a friend, or under the guidance of a trainer?

Certainly the home venue offers the advantages of privacy, twenty-four-hour access, and convenience, not to mention that it's less expensive. Training in the home with the Slow Burn at Home regimen is a great way for people to begin to reap the advantages of Slow Burn and to get their feet wet, so to speak, without making a big investment. Many of the at Home exercises also work well for those people who spend much of their time on the road and may not have access to weights or a gym. The downside of home training, in most instances, is the equipment—or, more specifically, the lack of it. Consequently, we designed the at Home regimen to accommodate the majority of people, who fall into the don't-have-machines-at-home category. This regimen relies on using your own weight, a few simple training tools, and a few small weights, all of which you can fashion from things you probably have around the house. If you have never done any strength training and want to wade in slowly, it's a good place to begin; make no mistake, there are plenty of gains you can make in strength, flexibility, and conditioning without ever leaving the privacy of your home. If you happen to be fortunate enough to have a multifunction machine, a set of free weights and benches, or a full gym at your home, you can follow the Slow Burn in the Gym routine there and have the best of both worlds.

To reap the maximum rewards from Slow Burn, over the long haul, there's no doubt that a gym setting works best. If you have access to a gym, the YMCA, or a local fitness center where you can use machines and weights, you'll find it much easier to continually challenge yourself, and you will progress much faster.

Taking it even a step further, you may want to enlist the aid of a certified trainer to guide your progress; if you can find a Slow Burn Center or certified slow strength trainer nearby, so much the better. Although sessions with a trainer will cost you, you may want to sign up for just a few sessions, especially if you're new to strength training. A qualified professional will not only be able to instruct you on the proper use of the available machines and the correct form for each exercise, but will be better able to gauge when to challenge you with more weight or add additional exercises to your regimen. Availing yourself of a good strength trainer takes a lot of the guesswork out of strength training.

The choice is yours; it should suit you, your lifestyle, and your budget. But whatever venue works best for you, when you decide to join the Slow Burn Fitness Revolution, a stronger, leaner, healthier you is just thirty minutes a week away.

Slow Burn at Home

CHAPTER 9

The art of life is the avoiding of pain.

—THOMAS JEFFERSON

I f you've decided to begin by working at home, here's how you get started. In this chapter, you'll learn how to become leaner, healthier, and stronger in just thirty minutes a week, without ever leaving the comfort of your home or office. And what's more, to use the Slow Burn at Home regimen, you won't need to invest in any expensive equipment, although a few simple and inexpensive supplies will come in handy. For the most part, you'll only need items you already have around the house.

Gathering Some Simple Equipment

To perform your Slow Burn routine at home or in your office, you'll want to assemble these items:

- *Three bath towels, or two towels and an exercise mat*
  You'll be performing some of your exercises on the floor, and you'll want a mat or towel for comfort. In addition, you'll be using a couple of towels to make a low-back support roll for one of the exercises. They needn't be expensive towels; any towel will do, as long as it's a long (bath-sized) one.

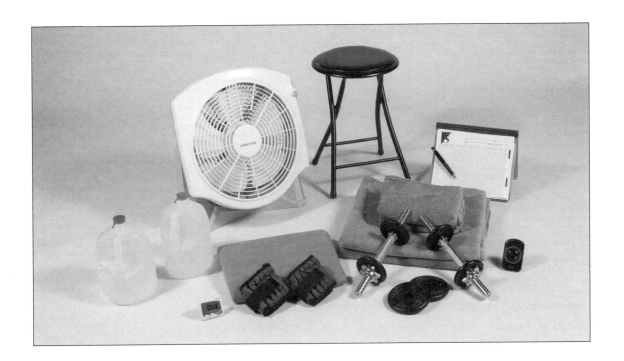

- *A sturdy stool the height of a chair seat, with or without a back, or a sturdy chair without arms.*

  You'll use the stool to sit on for certain exercises and as a support for others. A sturdy wooden or metal stool or bench will work best, but even a sturdy plastic stool is fine.

- *Adjustable dumbbells or a small set of hand weights ranging from two pounds to fifteen pounds or two plastic water or milk jugs with handles (marked in half-pound increments.)[1]*

[1]To mark the half-pound increments on the gallon jugs, fill each jug with about one cup of water and weigh it on a kitchen scale. It should weigh about half a pound. Adjust the water level slightly if needed and mark the water line with a permanent marker. Add another cup, weigh, and adjust as needed, and mark the line. Continue to add water in half-pound increments until you reach 5 or 6 pounds. A full gallon of water weighs about 8.3 pounds.

You can usually find inexpensive dumbbells in a variety of sizes in the sporting goods section of any discount store or on the Web; however, we've also included some exercise equipment resources in Appendix A. You'll note as you go through the exercises that beginning with just a pair of two- or three-pound dumbbells or hand weights and a five-pound pair will probably be fine for a start. And you can even be creative and make your own weights with quart, half-gallon, or gallon water or milk jugs filled with water, or even use cans of vegetables.

■ *A set of ankle weights that you can vary by the pound*

Like the dumbbells, simple ankle weights can be found in the sporting goods section of any big discount store or on the Web (or by using the resource list in Appendix A). You can even make a homemade ankle weight by using two quart-sized zip-closure bags filled with water, tightly sealed. A quart of water (four cups) weighs a touch over two pounds. You can affix the zip-closure ankle weight to your ankle with a piece of elastic bandage or even with duct tape if push comes to shove. If keeping cost to the bare minimum is important for you, be creative. You'll be amazed at what you can do.

■ *An inexpensive metronome*

A metronome is a wind-up, battery-powered, or plug-in device that is used to keep a steady beat and can be found at most music stores. While this may seem like an un-usual piece of equipment for a strength-training work-out, for the Slow Burn regimen, it's an important one. To properly perform Slow Burn, you must maintain a con-stant one-beat-per-second rhythm as you lift and lower the weights.

■ *A small fan (one you can easily move around as needed)*

To achieve the optimum results from your Slow Burn routine, you should avoid becoming overheated as you work.[2] This should be a no-sweat regimen, so we encourage you to keep the breeze moving with your portable fan.

- *A digital timer that can count down and beep*

  A really inexpensive one will do, if you don't already have one in your kitchen. We want you to spend no more than about ninety seconds performing each exercise perfectly with the proper weight. The Slow Burn program is about building health and fitness by taking your muscle groups, one by one, to utter fatigue. Once you learn the technique, it shouldn't take you more than ninety seconds to get there. The timer will keep you on track.

- *A record-keeping card and pencil (not a pen!) to record your progress*

  Accurate records will make tailoring your Slow Burn regimen to your specific needs infinitely easier. We've included a sample form in Appendix B for you to copy. Copy it and use it; you'll be glad you did!

Setting Up Your Slow Burn Work Space

Now that you've gathered your simple muscle-building equipment, you're ready to set up your training environment. Just as with any project that depends on focusing your concentration for maximum success, you'll want to create a work space for getting fit that fosters your ability to concentrate on the task at hand. This means eliminating as many distractions as possible. Turn off the TV, radio, or stereo, put

[2]Mildly warming the muscles allows the metabolic enzymes to function optimally. Overheating can hamper their function—thus the benefit of keeping cool with a fan and loose clothing during the workout.

out the dog, take the phone off the hook or send your calls to voice mail, close the door to the room.

Have the equipment you've gathered easily accessible and at the ready. Dress in comfortable, cool clothing. Place the fan in a spot that will keep the air circulating around you, cooling you while you work.

Timing Is Everything

To set the rhythm of the workout, turn on your metronome and adjust it to sixty beats per minute (BPM), giving you a one-beat-per-second constant rhythm at which to work. When you're ready to begin your workout, you will set the timer, usually to 100 seconds.

The 100-second interval will give you:

- Ten seconds, or beats of the metronome, to get into position, settled, and ready
- Twenty to thirty seconds, or beats, to complete each of the three repetitions, including
  - Three full beats to initiate movement and to move the first inch
  - Seven full beats (at least) to complete the lifting phase, moving about one inch per beat
  - Three full beats to reverse direction and move the first inch of the return
  - Seven full beats (at least) to complete the return, moving about one inch per beat.

If you are still exercising when the timer beeps—i.e., if you could continue doing repetitions in good form—the weight is too light, and you'll need to increase it or change the exercise position to a more advanced one. (You'll find these advanced positions in the "Tailoring Your Routine" section following each exercise.)

On your progress card, you'll want to note in seconds the time it takes you to reach muscle failure for each exercise. For instance, if on Monday you do an exercise and reach muscle fatigue in seventy seconds, you will note this on your card. Perhaps the next time you do that exercise, say on the following Friday, you reach fatigue in eighty-eight seconds. That's great improvement, and it's time for you to bump up the resistance or try a harder position for that exercise. It's helpful to see consistent progress, and that's why it's important to note the time it takes you to reach complete muscle fatigue each time you do an exercise.

Some Important Safety Tips Before You Begin

- Breathe freely at all times. Never hold your breath. How you breathe is less important than breathing freely throughout the duration of the exercise.
- Keep your hands loose whenever possible; gripping your hands tightly can elevate your blood pressure.
- Relax your face and jaw, even letting your lips part slightly. Keep a steady head and neck position, with your chin slightly tucked in as though you were trying to hold an orange under it. Don't crane your neck backward or twist it from side to side.
- Dress in cool, comfortable clothing, so that you don't overheat. Sweating is a sign of overheating. Use that fan!
- Always favor perfect form—slow, controlled speed, good body mechanics, relaxed breathing, correct timing—over recorded time, number of reps, or the amount of weight

you lift. Injuries occur when you strain, twist, or jerk trying to lift too much, go too fast, or do too many repetitions. Remember that your true goal with every exercise is to reach the deepest level of muscle fatigue in perfect form. Trying to perform as many repetitions as you can, any way you can, is a false goal. Rely on intellect over instinct always!

- If you experience a headache while exercising, **stop immediately and rest** until the headache goes away completely; never, never continue to exercise.

- You may feel a slight burning sensation in your muscles during the exercises; this is not an indication to stop, unless, of course, it becomes severe. Continue the exercise until you truly cannot go on moving your limbs in good, slow, careful form. Assuming that you fatigue in the target time (sixty to ninety seconds), this ensures that you have reached a level of intensity that will stimulate increases in strength. But if you feel pain in your joints, especially a sharp, sudden pain, this is an indication that something is amiss. You should stop the exercise and, if the pain persists, seek the advice of a physician.

Getting with the Slow Burn Program

When you're ready to begin your workout, get your progress chart and pencil ready. Date the progress record and make sure to record the specifics of your routine after each exercise or you'll forget. Knowing what you've done well will dictate when it's time to move ahead and challenge yourself a little more. Your recorded progress is an invaluable tool for success.

To make your first session run more smoothly, read the instructions for each of the exercises carefully, going over them a few times and referring to the pictures before you're ready to begin. That way, you'll be familiar with correct form, timing, and posture from the get-go.

And finally, remember that the Slow Burn workout is tough but short, and infinitely profitable to your health. Strength training is not supposed to entertain you; it's not necessarily even supposed to be enjoyable. That's the difference between exercising and engaging in a leisure activity. A Slow Burn workout will give you maximum benefits in terms of strength gain, improved cardiovascular and metabolic fitness, increased flexibility, and better health in the shortest amount of time. You can make it the most effective and productive twenty-five to thirty minutes of your week.

The Slow Burn at Home Routine

Now, let's take a look at the exercises that make up your total-fitness workouts. Each specific exercise works a group of related muscles; the routine, as a whole, strengthens just about every muscle in your body, either directly or indirectly. You'll want to perform the routine in the order we've outlined below to reap the maximum benefit from your Slow Burn program.

EXERCISE		MUSCLES WORKED
#1	Push-ups	Chest, arms, shoulders
#2	Doorknob squats	Buttocks, thighs
#3	Side-lying leg lifts	Buttocks (sides)
#4	Single-leg curls	Rear thighs, calves
#5	Side-shoulder raise	Shoulders
#6	Overhead press	Shoulders, arms, neck

Exercise	Muscles Worked
#7 Single-arm back pull-ups	Back, upper arms
#8 Biceps curls	Upper arms
#9 Shoulder shrugs	Upper neck, shoulders
#10 Abdominal crunches	Abdominal muscles
#11 Heel raises	Calves (lower leg)

Familiarize yourself with each of the exercises before you begin. You may even want to try just a couple of them at first to get the hang of this very slow, focused, deliberate style of exercising. Once you're comfortable with how to do each of them, you're ready to begin your journey to better health, greater strength, and improved fitness in just twenty-five to thirty minutes a week!

#1 Push-ups

GET READY

Tools you'll need: 3 towels

You'll need your towels for this exercise. Fold each of the towels into a square. Place one on the floor in front of you, where your forehead will touch the ground, and the other two under your knees.

Set your timer to 100 seconds (10 seconds to get into position and 90 seconds to complete the exercise).

GET SET

Kneel down on the towels and then place your hands, shoulder's width apart, on the floor in front of you in line with your armpits. Hold your body weight steady in the start position with elbows locked straight and back straight (no swaybacked mules or arched alley cats allowed). Your feet can either touch the ground lightly or stay elevated. Keep your chin tucked in a bit, so you're not tempted to crane your neck backward. Pretend you're holding a tennis ball between your chin and chest. This posture will lengthen and straighten your neck and prevent injury.

GO!

- Be sure to maintain relaxed, even breathing throughout. Do not hold your breath, clench your teeth, grimace, or strain.
- SLOWLY, taking at least 3 seconds or beats of the metronome to lower yourself the first inch, descend smoothly until your forehead reaches the towel. Take a minimum of 7 full beats to get the rest of the way down. Now, careful! When your forehead reaches the towel, reverse direction extremely slowly without resting. Take no more than the briefest pause there before reversing directions.
- Again take 3 full beats to move the first inch as you push back up, moving 1 inch per second. Continue pressing your body upward until you are at the straight-arm position, but *do not lock* your elbows. You've just completed one repetition. Count it out: say "One" out loud.
- SLOWLY reverse direction again, taking the full 3-beat count to descend the first inch and then a full 7 beats to reach the ground, trying to smoothly move just 1 inch per beat. Pause briefly and reverse slowly, taking 3 full beats to begin your upward press, and 7 full beats to almost reach the straight-arm position. This is the completion of your second rep; say "Two" out loud.
- If you're able, reverse, and complete another rep, counting it out. Continue until

you honestly cannot go on. When your forehead touches the towel and your arms can no longer press upward to lift your forehead from the towel (without breaking perfect form by jerking, thrusting, or resting), you've completed the exercise.

RELAX

At this point, slowly let your chest come down to the floor and rest there for a few seconds, but no more than 1 minute. Remember to continue your relaxed, even breathing all the while. Use your workout card to note your "time to failure" in seconds and the number of repetitions you completed or attempted to complete.

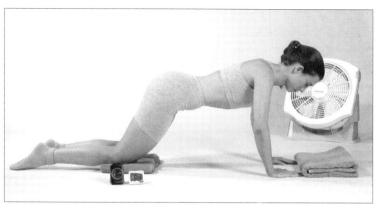

START

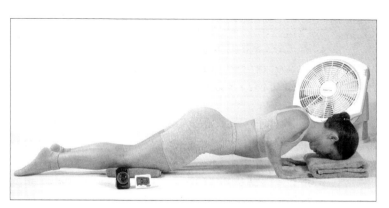

FINISH

Tailoring your routine . . .

If you were able to take the muscles of your arms, chest, and shoulders to complete failure in 3 repetitions within the 90-second interval, congratulations! This level of intensity is just right for you. However, with any strength routine, it would be unusual to hit the perfect blend of timing and effort on the first go. So, don't fret if you didn't. To refine your routine, take a look at these commonly voiced concerns and the adjustments you can make to keep the Slow Burn system working most effectively for you.

"I'm too weak to do even one push-up!"
If you're not strong enough to raise your body even once, begin by just doing the lowering part of the exercise. Once your forehead touches the towel, carefully sit back on your heels and then push up and forward to return to the starting position. Immediately get set and slowly begin to descend again. Continue to perform the lowering half of the push-up until you cannot lower your body with complete control, in perfect form. In time, this technique will strengthen your arms, chest, and shoulders enough for you to do the full Slow Burn push-up.

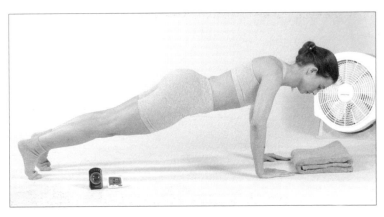

START

"I'm too strong; I'm able to continue my slow repetitions without reaching total fatigue, even after 120 seconds."

If you are already too strong to reach fatigue by the 120-second mark, you're ready for a more advanced posture. Instead of starting from the knees, begin with your toes on the floor, your body fully straight and supported on your arms and toes. You can put away those knee towels. We want to warn you, however, that performed precisely as described and in perfect form, this advanced technique is very difficult. Without momentum to propel you up and down, don't be surprised if your arms fatigue after only a few reps—even if you're used to doing many "standard" push-ups. Don't equate what you did the old way with your new slow and focused approach. You may fatigue after a single rep done this way; if so, drop your knees and complete the exercise that way. Soon you'll be able to add more reps in the advanced posture. Or check out the following tip.

"I'm too strong for the beginner knee push-ups but too weak for even one advanced one!"

In that case, begin on your toes and lower yourself to the bottom in the advanced posture, then drop your knees and slowly begin to push back up from the less advanced knee posture. At the starting point, again straighten your knees, supporting your weight on toes and arms, and lower yourself in the advanced posture. Continue until you cannot raise your forehead from the towel or until you cannot lower yourself in good form.

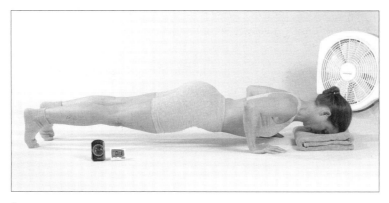

FINISH

#2 Doorknob Squats

GET READY

Tools you'll need: a stool and a door with knobs

Open the door halfway, so that you can grab both doorknobs. Even though your arms feel like spaghetti from the push-ups, don't rest. Place the stool about 2 feet from the edge of the door. Adjust the fan, if needed, so that it blows on your body, but not in your eyes; watering eyes will break your concentration. You're about to begin the most difficult of the Slow Burn home exercises—squats—and performing them perfectly will require total focus.

Set your timer to 100 seconds.

GET SET

Lightly grasp both doorknobs at arm's length with an underhand grip—that is, with your palms facing the ceiling. Position yourself at the edge of the door, feet apart and

to either side of it, with your own "seat" centered over the seat of the stool. Keep your feet slightly in front of your knees to avoid putting undue pressure on the knees. Holding the doorknobs at arm's length will help keep your knees in the proper position at least an inch or so behind your toes.

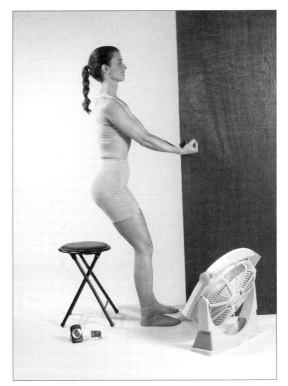

START

Go!

- Keep your breathing easy and relaxed throughout the exercise. Never hold your breath, grit your teeth, or grimace. Be careful not to pull yourself up using the strength of your arms (although they're probably still pretty spent from the push-ups); your light touch on the doorknobs is for balance and safety only. Keep your focus on the muscles of your buttocks and thighs as they move smoothly through the exercise.

- Holding lightly to the doorknobs for balance, SLOWLY begin to lower your body, keeping your knees behind your toes, taking a full 3 beats to initiate the downward movement. Continue, smoothly lowering yourself about 1 inch per beat, until your rear end touches the stool. Take a full 7 beats to complete the lowering phase. Pause briefly, but *do not sit and rest*.

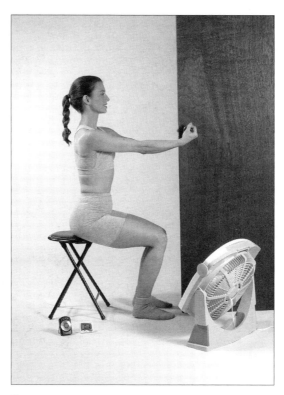

FINISH

- As soon as your rear end lightly touches the stool, take at least 3 beats to initiate a slow and careful reverse of direction, pushing mainly through your heels. Do not let your heels come off the floor. Then take a full 7 beats to complete the rising phase to return to the standing position. Don't completely straighten your legs or lock your knees (this will stop the muscle work). Stop rising when you feel the exercise becoming easy on your muscles; pause and reverse direction to keep your muscles working. You've completed 1 rep; count it out as "One," but keep your focus.
- Again, take the full 3 beats to pause, reverse direction, and begin to lower yourself again, trying to smoothly move about an inch per beat. Lightly touch the stool, pause for a whisper of a second, then take 3 full beats to reverse direction and slowly and smoothly rise again to the near-standing position at the 1-inch-per-beat speed. That's rep number 2; count it out loud as "Two," but keep your focus.
- Continue the squat repetitions until you truly cannot rise from the stool again.

RELAX

Give yourself the briefest moment here to breathe and relax, but move on as quickly as you possibly can to Exercise #3, Side-Lying Leg Lifts. Remember the number of reps and your time to failure, so that you can record them on your workout card after you complete the next exercise.

Tailoring your routine . . .

"I can't even rise up off the stool once!"
That's okay, just do the lowering part of the exercise at first and use your arms to pull yourself back up. Be sure to still initiate the lowering slowly over the full 3 beats and take the full 7 seconds to descend. Don't sit and rest, but simply assist your rise with your arm strength. Before too long, you'll be able to depend less and less on your arms, and finally, you'll be able to do it all with your buttock and leg strength alone.

"It seems too easy. I can already continue to perform squats even past the 120-second mark."
Really?! Properly performed, Slow Burn squats are tough. First, check that you've properly set your metronome at 60 beats per minute (or 1 beat per second). Next, be sure you're taking 3 full beats to initiate the downward motion, moving no faster than 1 inch per second, that you're taking 7 full beats to lower to the stool, a full 3 beats to

pause and reverse direction, and a full 7 beats to make your ascent. Check to see that you're neither resting on the stool at the bottom nor taking the load off your muscles by standing too straight or locking your knees at the top. Make certain you're not assisting your rise with arm strength—keep just a light touch on the doorknobs. If you're sure you are performing the exercise with proper timing and form, you are indeed strong enough for a more advanced technique: Remove the stool.

Now, from the same starting position, lower yourself slowly until the backs of your thighs just touch your calves or come close, pause for an instant, then slowly reverse direction to rise again. Remember not to assist with your arms and to rise only to the point at which you feel the exercise becoming easier, then pause and reverse from there. If you need to challenge your muscles even further, instead of the customary 7 beats, move even more slowly: take 10 or 15 seconds to lower and 10 or 15 to rise up.

#3 Side-Lying Leg Lifts

GET READY

Tools you'll need: ankle weights (optional) and a towel or mat

Depending on your buttock and hip strength, you may need the ankle weights for this one. Try the routine without them at first and see if you can reach the 2-minute mark using only the weight of your own leg. If the weight of your leg is too light, add the ankle weights. And don't forget that since you'll be working just one leg at a time, you can even use both ankle weights on one ankle as your strength increases.

Set your timer for 100 seconds.

GET SET

Place the towel or mat on the floor, positioned under your hip. Lie on your right side, resting your head on your right hand and bent right arm as shown. Keep your hips and shoulders in line with each other and perpendicular to the floor throughout the exercise. Bend your right leg slightly at the knee. Place your left palm on the floor in front of your chest for support and to prevent your body from rocking forward. Keep your left (working) leg straight and slightly behind the right one.

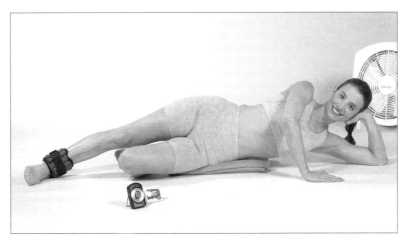

START

Go!

- Breathe in a relaxed, even fashion throughout the exercise. Never hold your breath, grunt, grimace, or clench your teeth.

- Take a full 3 beats to initiate the lifting movement of your working leg. As slowly as possible, moving no faster than 1 inch per beat, try to smoothly raise your working leg off the floor as high as possible without arching or contorting your back. Take the full 7-beat count to complete the lift if you can, focusing on the work you're doing with only the muscles in the side of your buttock and hip.

- Pause for a few beats at your high point to squeeze the hip/buttock muscle. Then, slowly reverse direction over 3 beats and again try taking the full 7 beats to smoothly lower your leg until the inner thigh of your working leg just lightly touches your other thigh.

- Without a second of rest, take 3 full beats to reverse direction and once again begin raising your leg as slowly as possible, trying to keep your speed at no more than 1 inch per beat. Remember to breathe.

- Pause at the high point to squeeze the buttock and hip muscles, then slowly reverse direction and lower again to just touch the thighs together.

- Continue these repetitions in good form until you honestly cannot raise your working leg again.

- Sit up on your towel or mat, extend both legs in front of you, bent slightly at the knee, and "shake out" the muscles of your thigh for a few seconds. Reset your timer for 100 seconds, quickly roll to your left side, and get into the starting position to work your right leg in exactly the same manner. Note your reps and time on your workout card.

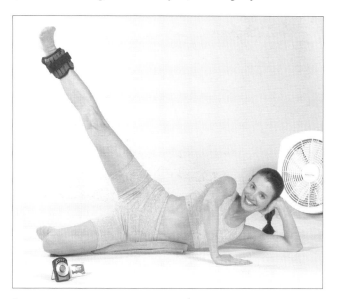

FINISH

"I'm so stiff; I can't raise my leg very high at all."
Don't worry. There's no preset height requirement that you must meet. You'll be doing
plenty of muscle work all the same. All that's necessary is that you go as high as you
comfortably can each time you do the exercise. As you become stronger, you'll find
that you'll be able to take your leg higher and higher. Often, the restriction in motion
you see in the beginning isn't from stiffness of the joints or tightness of the ligaments
supporting them as much as from weakness in the muscles moving them. Keep at it
and you'll see an improvement in your range of motion.

"It's too easy for me. I can easily lift my leg and lower it past the 90-second mark."
Make sure you're not going too fast and using momentum to make the work easier or
assisting the lift by pushing on the floor with your hand, rather than using just the focused effort of the muscles in the side of the buttock and hip. If indeed you are not,
then you need the increased challenge of adding weight to your working leg. First add
one ankle weight, and if that's still too easy add a second—and even a third if you're
really strong.

#4 Single-Leg Curls

GET READY

Tools you'll need: a stool and one ankle weight

Start with 5 pounds. This will probably be too light, but give it a try.

Set your timer to 100 seconds.

GET SET

To begin, place the ankle weight securely on one ankle, so it doesn't slip up your leg toward your knee when you do the exercise. Set the stool in front of you and place both hands on it. Keeping your back straight, lean forward at a slight angle. Keep your exercising knee slightly bent at the start.

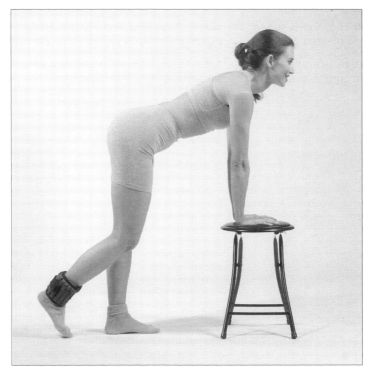

START

Go!

- Breathe in a relaxed, even fashion. Refrain from holding your breath, grimacing, grunting, or clenching your teeth.

- Slowly, taking 3 full beats to initiate the first inch of movement, begin to bend your knee. Keep your ankle flexed (toes pointed toward your knee) and your opposite leg completely straight. Bend your knee until your heel comes as close to your buttocks as possible in a minimum of 7 more full beats, longer if possible.

- Pause and squeeze the muscles in the back of your thigh as hard as you can, but be careful not to cramp your leg. Slowly reverse direction, taking a full 3 beats to do so, then try to take at least 7 beats to return to your starting position, with your toes lightly touching the ground.

- Without a second of rest, reverse direction again, taking at least 3 full seconds to move 1 inch, and then continuing as slowly as possible. Remember to keep breathing.

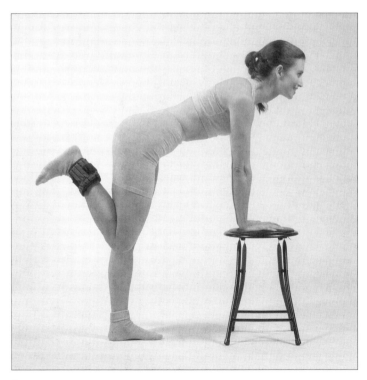

Finish

- Keep going in this fashion until you honestly cannot continue to bend your knee in good form.
- Once you've reached complete muscle fatigue (remember, that's your success end-point), place the ankle weight on the other leg and work it in the same manner. Note the time to failure and your reps on your workout card.

Tailoring your routine . . .

"It's just too easy. I could go on forever."
Try doubling up on the ankle weights. Put both on one leg and give that a try. Eventually you may even want to purchase heavier ankle weights.

Now, let's give your tired lower body a bit of a rest and do some more work on the upper body.

#5 Side-Shoulder Raise and #6 Overhead Press

GET READY

Tools you'll need: a stool and dumbbells or water jugs

To begin, try using the 5-pound weights or filled water jugs at first and from there experiment with heavier or lighter weights. Remember, what you're seeking is a weight that you can lift correctly using perfect form for 3, or at most 4, repetitions before totally fatiguing the working muscles. It's not a contest to see how much weight you can lift. It's a journey to take your muscle to success through failure with the correct movement and the correct weight.

Adjust the position of your fan if necessary and set the timer for 100 seconds.

GET SET

Place the dumbbells or jugs on either side of you as you sit down on the stool with your knees together and your feet in front of you. Bend down and grasp the weights, letting them hang dead at your sides. Sit up tall, straight, and relaxed; try not to lean back or tip forward when doing the exercise. Keep your torso from swaying to and fro or leaning from side to side.

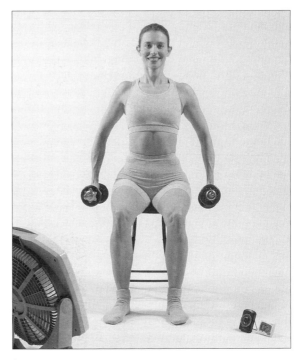

START

Go!

- Breathe in a relaxed, even fashion throughout the exercise. Never hold your breath, clench your teeth, grimace, or strain. Focus on the muscles of your shoulders and upper arms as they smoothly work.
- Slowly initiate the lifting movement, raising the weights away from your sides for 3 beats of the metronome, then continue to smoothly lift the weight, moving 1 inch per beat, until your arms are parallel with the ground or slightly higher, taking 7 full beats to complete the movement.
- Pause in this position for 2 to 3 beats, then slowly (3 beats) begin to reverse direction and, moving at 1 inch per beat, slowly lower the weight. Remember, take 7 full beats to lower the weights smoothly to a point about 1 inch away from your hips (don't let them touch).
- Let the weights hover 1 inch from your hips for a second and then slowly reverse direction and begin to lift through the 7-beat interval again.
- Continue smoothly lifting and lowering until you cannot raise the weights away from your sides but DO NOT REST . . . move to the Overhead Press right away. (Note: For this exercise, you won't use the timer. Instead, just count repetitions.)

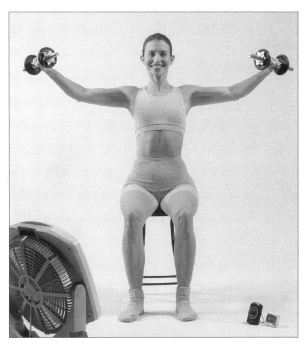

FINISH

- IMMEDIATELY, but smoothly, bring the weights to shoulder height, and once there, SLOWLY initiate movement by pressing them overhead. Be sure to keep the dumbbells or jugs slightly in front of your face. Take the full 7 beats to complete the rising phase of the exercise, stopping just short of fully straightening your arms—*do not lock your elbows!!* (Locking the joints will shift the work of supporting the weight from your muscles, where you want it, to your bones.)

- At the top of the lift, pause briefly, then slowly reverse direction and begin to lower the weights to shoulder level again over the full 7-beat interval. Do not rest the weights on your shoulders, but rather pause briefly and reverse direction to begin another lift if you're able.

- Continue lifting and lowering—7 beats up, 3 to reverse, and 7 down—until you can no longer raise the weights from shoulder level. Record the number of repetitions. If you can complete more than 6 reps, maintaining perfect form and timing, the weight is too light and you should increase by half a pound to 1 pound. Don't forget to record your reps and your time getting to the success-through-failure endpoint on your card.

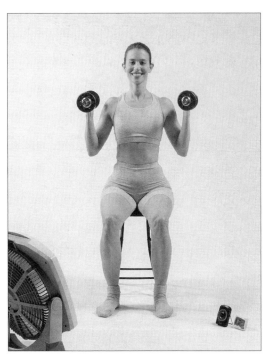

START

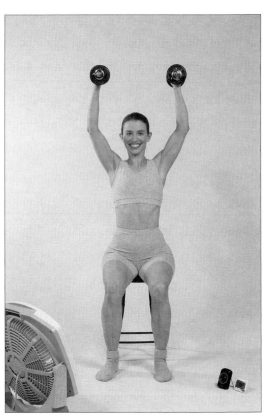

FINISH

RELAX

Slowly return the weights to the floor and allow your arms and shoulders to relax. Take a few smooth, deep breaths to unwind.

Tailoring your routine . . .

"My elbows hurt just a bit when I do the side raises."
As long as it's just a bit, this isn't an uncommon complaint at first, and you can usually solve the problem by keeping your elbows slightly bent when you do the exercise.

"The weight I use for side raises is too light for the overhead shoulder press."
That one's easy to fix. Just place a pair of heavier dumbbells next to the stool at the start. When you reach the success-through-failure point with the side raises, return those weights to the floor, smoothly pick up the heavier dumbbells, bring them to shoulder level, and begin the Overhead Press. Remember, it's critical that you not rest for even 5 seconds between the Side-Shoulder Raise and the Overhead Press, so strive to make this transition fluid and efficient. Bear in mind, too, that you may have to experiment a bit to find the perfect weight for each exercise, but in time you will. Finding that perfect resistance is yet another reason to keep a clear and accurate record of your progress (and one of the great values of a good instructor, too!).

#7 Single-Arm Back Pull-ups

GET READY

Tools you'll need: a stool and a 6- to 8-pound dumbbell or filled gallon jug of water.

In this exercise, you'll be working one arm at a time; the other will support and stabilize your torso. Place the stool where it's stable and you've got room to work. Adjust the position of the fan if necessary so that it will keep you cool but not blow directly in your face. Set your timer to 100 seconds.

GET SET

Stand facing the stool, with one foot forward and your legs comfortably apart at about shoulder's width, so you'll have a strong, stable foundation. Place one hand on the stool as your support hand. It should be your left one if you've got your left foot forward, your

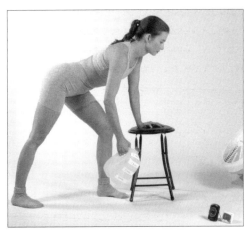

START

right one if your right foot is forward. Lean forward toward the stool at about a 45-degree angle and arch your back like an alley cat, but very slightly. Take the dumbbell or water jug in your working hand and let the weight hang dead beside the stool.

GO!

- Breathe in a relaxed and even fashion throughout the exercise. Do not hold your breath, clench your teeth, grunt, grimace, or strain. Focus on the muscles of your back and upper arm as they work smoothly through the movement.
- Slowly initiate the movement of pulling the dumbbell back and upward beside you, taking 3 full beats to move the first inch. Continue to smoothly raise the weight, moving about 1 inch per beat, using only the target muscle groups, until your hand reaches the chest/armpit level.
- Pause here briefly, squeezing your arm and back muscles for a few beats as you think: *"I will make my elbow touch the ceiling."*
- Reverse direction slowly (over a 3-beat interval) and begin to lower the weight just as slowly until your arm is almost completely straight. Maintain the resistance on the muscle groups at this lower point by keeping just a slight bend in your elbow. *Don't rest your arm in a straight position and let the weight hang.*

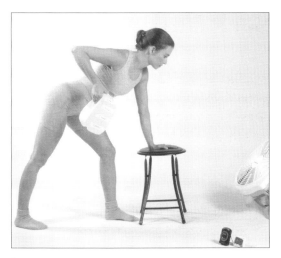

FINISH

- IMMEDIATELY, without pause, initiate the slow reverse of direction and begin again to pull the weight up 1 inch per second until it reaches armpit/chest level and you mentally aim your elbow toward the ceiling.
- Pause again, squeezing your arm and back muscles, envisioning your elbow touching the ceiling, then reverse and lower just as slowly to the slightly bent lower position.
- Continue lifting and lowering until you cannot lift the weight another time and still maintain perfect form and timing. If you would have to grunt, strain, jerk, or lean in order to continue, you've reached the success-through-failure endpoint.
- Now switch to the other side and repeat this process. Don't be alarmed if your new support arm (the one you just worked) feels like a piece of overcooked spaghetti. That's normal and not a problem, as long as it can safely support you. Be sure to record your reps and your time on your chart.

Tailoring your routine . . .

"When I switch to the other side my exercised arm shakes like a leaf!"
Excellent! This reaction simply means you worked your muscles hard enough to stimulate a strengthening response—that's exactly what you're trying to do. After a time, the shaking will subside a bit and you'll get used to it. But if you're shaking so much that you feel you will lose your balance, wait 3 minutes before starting the exercise with your other arm. That brief rest will allow you to replenish your energy sufficiently to stay stable as you work but will not interfere with the rhythm of the routine.

"I can't lift the plastic jug full of water even once!"
Remember, your jug should be marked in half-pound increments. Pour out some water—maybe a pound—and try it again. If it's still too heavy, keep emptying water until you can complete at least one full repetition. Or try using a 14-ounce or 15-ounce can of vegetables as a substitute dumbbell.

#8 Biceps Curls

GET READY

Tools you'll need: a stool and dumbbells or filled gallon jugs of water

Now that the back pull-ups have exhausted your biceps somewhat, you're ready to more completely fatigue the muscles of your upper arms and forearms. Begin with about 5 pounds of weight and adjust up or down as needed to reach success through failure within the 90-second interval. Set your timer for 100 seconds and . . .

GET SET

Sit on the stool with good posture, take a dumbbell or jug in each hand, and let the weights hang down on either side of your knees, arms extended and elbows slightly bent. Tuck your elbows into your sides, *where they should stay for the duration of this exercise!* Pretend your arms above the elbow are glued to your sides. Don't let your upper arms drift away from your sides or sway to and fro. Keep your spine erect and your torso still—no leaning or swaying backward and forward. The only thing that should move is your lower arm, as it smoothly and slowly bends and unbends. Focus on the muscles of your upper arm (your biceps) and your forearm as they do all the work.

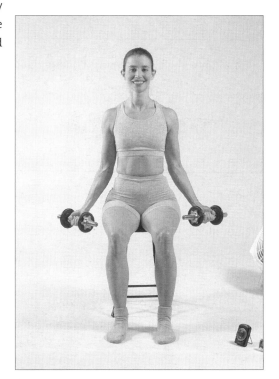

START

Go!

- Breathe in a relaxed, even fashion throughout the exercise. No holding your breath, gritting your teeth, grunting, grimacing, or straining allowed.
- Slowly initiate the movement of bending your elbows to lift the dumbbell, taking 3 full beats of the metronome to do it. Keep the lifting motion slow and deliberate, moving 1 inch per second, and taking the full 7 beats to complete the lifting phase of the exercise. As you lift, allow your wrists to naturally flex or curl inward slightly, as if you were trying to touch your shoulders with your knuckles; this will benefit your forearms.
- Pause when you've brought your hands as close as possible to your body, and briefly (2 or 3 beats) squeeze the muscles of your upper arm and forearm. *Do not allow your arms to rise to a position fully perpendicular to the ground.* (Doing so will unload the weight from your muscles and make the exercise less effective.)
- Now, take a full 3 beats to reverse direction and begin to slowly lower the weights (over 7 full beats), uncurling your wrists as the weights get to waist level and stopping when your arms are extended but still slightly flexed at the elbows.

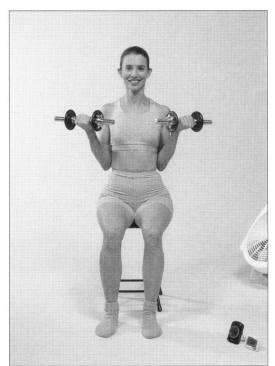

- Pause at the low point, slowly reverse direction, and begin the 7-beat lifting interval once again.
- Continue to the success-through-failure endpoint, when you can no longer lower the weights smoothly and/or cannot lift them again. Record your time and reps in your progress chart.

Relax

Slowly rise from the stool and take a few deep, satisfied breaths ... you're in the home stretch now!

Finish

9 Shoulder Shrugs

GET READY

Tools you'll need: a stool and completely filled water jugs or 10-pound dumbbells.
   Set your timer to 100 seconds.

GET SET

Place the water jugs or weights on either side of the stool. Sit on the stool and lean
forward to grab one in each hand. Slowly come to an upright sitting position. Let the
weights hang from your sides, slightly away from your hips. You should feel a good
stretch in the upper neck and shoulders.

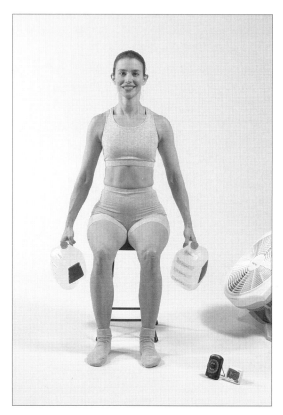

START

Go!

- Breathe in a relaxed, even fashion. Don't hold your breath, grimace, grunt, or contort your face. Stay focused on the muscles of your upper neck and shoulders.
- Slowly, taking 3 full beats to initiate the movement, raise the tops of your shoulders up as if to touch the edges of your shoulders to your earlobes in a minimum of 7 beats, as if you were saying to someone, "I don't know," but in very slow motion.
- Pause, squeezing the muscles of your upper neck and shoulders for a full 3 beats, then reverse direction and slowly lower in a minimum of 7 beats.
- Once you reach your starting position, reverse slowly and repeat until you reach muscle fatigue and cannot raise the weights up again in good form. Remember not to slouch forward or lean backward; keep sitting upright. Don't bend your elbows, either—keep them straight.

Tailoring your routine . . .

"I feel deep tension in my neck doing this exercise. Is this okay?"

You bet it is! This tension is the very stimulus needed to create stronger neck muscles. If your neck muscles get sore, don't worry; after a time, the soreness will subside. Sharp or severe pain is another matter. You should stop any exercise if you feel sudden sharp pain.

FINISH

#10 Abdominal Crunches

GET READY

Tools you'll need: 3 towels (or a mat and 2 towels)

Place two towels on the floor, one on top of the other. Starting at one end, roll them up together lengthwise to make a soft, compact lower-back roll that is about 6 inches thick. You'll place this under the small of your lower back to give your abdominal muscles a slight stretch during their workout. Set your timer to 100 seconds and . . .

GET SET

Lie on your back on the third towel or your mat. Bend your knees at a 90-degree angle and position your feet flat on the mat or towel, a few inches apart. Hold your arms straight out, as if trying to touch your knees with your fingertips. Keep your chin tucked into your chest and focus your eyes on the center of your abdomen.

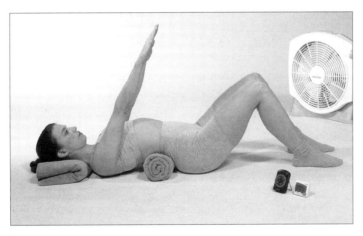

START

Go!

- Breathe in a relaxed and even fashion throughout the exercise. Do not hold your breath, clench your teeth, grunt, grimace, jerk, bounce, or strain at any time.

- Slowly begin to curl your torso upward and forward (taking a full 3 beats to move the first inch or two), as if trying to touch your knees with your fingertips. Focus your gaze at the center of your abdomen, as if a tractor beam were pulling you along that sight line at 1 inch per second. You're not trying to sit all the way up; only your shoulder blades should roll up and off the floor. Keep your lower back firmly in contact with the towel; if it raises up off the towel you have gone too far.

- Pause when your fingertips touch your knees or when they're as close as they can get, and focus hard on squeezing your abdominal muscles. Really tighten them; pretend Mike Tyson is about to punch you in the gut. Keep at it. Squeeeeeeezzzzze those muscles for 3 beats of the metronome and keep breathing in and out. This is a spot at which you're going to be tempted to strain and hold your breath. Fight that temptation for all you're worth.

- Now, SLOWLY lower your upper torso until your shoulder blades just touch the floor again, but *do not rest!* Try to take the full 7 counts to lower yourself if you can, but in any event, try to move no faster than 1 inch per second.

- Immediately initiate a reversal of direction and slowly begin to rise up again. With your fingertips, reach toward your knees, keep your lower back pinned to the towel, moving slowly and deliberately, 1 inch per second. Pause and squeeze your abdominal muscles tightly for 2 or 3 beats, reverse direction, and lower again to touch your shoulder blades to the floor for a whisper of a beat before reversing again.

- Continue to the success-through-failure endpoint where you can't possibly pull yourself up again. Record your reps and time on your progress chart.

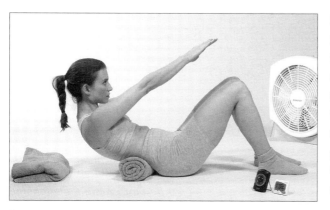

FINISH

Relax

Lie on your towel or mat for a few seconds; breathe deeply and slowly and just relax. Slowly sit up and then stand. Don't be surprised if you feel a little cramping in your abdominal muscles—you've just given them a terrific Slow Burn workout. Just take a few more deep breaths and relax.

Tailoring your routine . . .

"My abs are so weak, I can't do even one crunch!"
Don't fret—you're not alone. Properly done, these crunches are difficult, and you may need to assist your abdominal muscles at first. Here are two ways you can do that. First, try bringing your outstretched fingers a bit lower for the rising phase, so that you can touch your midthigh. Using your fingertips, crawl up your thigh as you crunch and let your arms assist in the lift. Pause and squeeze just as in the normal routine, then let your fingertips crawl back down to almost rest. If you still can't do the crunch, try this: Move over to the door, open it, and straddle it with your legs. Take another towel and wrap it around both doorknobs; use the towel to gently assist you in rising to the squeeze position. Then after pausing, try to lower slowly while holding the towel, but without using the strength of your arms. Eventually you will be able to do the crunches without using your arms at all.

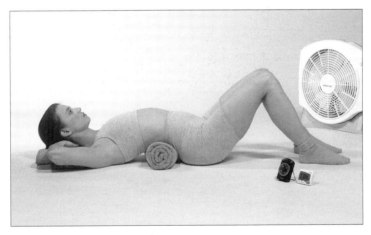

START (THE HARDER CRUNCH)

"The crunches are too easy; I can do these well past even the 90-second mark."
Is that so? Well, this time place your hands behind your head, arms relaxed and uninvolved in the work. Do the crunches this way until you get to the last one you can manage in this position, then very quickly switch to the arms-to-knees method and continue. When you reach success-through-failure using this easier method, hold the crunched position, put your hands back behind your head, and hold this advanced position until you cannot hold your body up anymore. Quite a bit harder, isn't it?

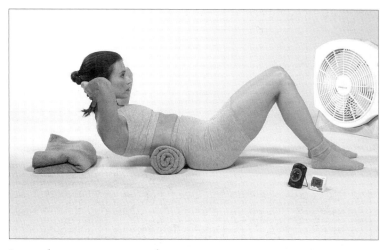

FINISH (THE HARDER CRUNCH)

#11 Heel Raises

GET READY

Tools you'll need: 2 towels

Set your timer for 100 seconds.

GET SET

Fold or roll the 2 towels. Place them side by side approximately 3 feet away from a wall. Step onto the towels, placing just the balls of your feet on them, with each foot at the center of a towel. Place your hands a shoulder's width apart against the wall. Straighten your arms completely, locking your elbows. Stand facing the wall, your feet a shoulder's width apart and parallel. Feel the good stretch in your calf muscles for a few seconds (it really does feel good). If you need to, move the towels back just a little farther to get a bit more stretch. You can also add to the stretch by bending your elbows slightly and bringing your chest closer to the wall.

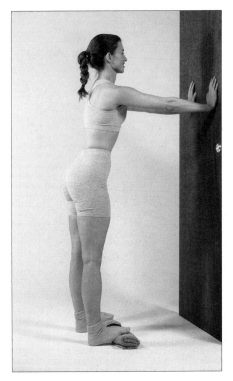

START

Go!

- Remember to breathe in a relaxed, even fashion throughout the exercise. Never hold your breath, grit your teeth, grunt, grimace, or strain.
- Slowly begin to raise your heels from the floor, taking a 3-beat interval to initiate the movement and move the first inch. Continue slowly and steadily rising about 1 inch per second until you're on your toes and the balls of your feet. Try to take the full 7 beats to complete the rising phase of the exercise. Focus on balancing almost completely on your big toes; *don't allow your feet to roll over onto your pinky toes.*
- Pause to squeeze the calf muscles of both legs for a few beats of the metronome, and then reverse direction and slowly begin to lower to the stretched position again over a 7-beat interval, letting your heels barely touch the floor before reversing direction and rising slowly again.
- Continue to slowly rise to your toes and lower almost to your heels until you've reached the success-through-failure endpoint—that is, when you cannot rise again with good form and timing. Be prepared for some soreness in your calf muscles tomorrow morning. That's normal, but will subside as you become stronger.

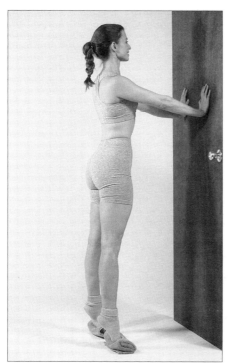

FINISH

Tailoring your routine . . .

"My body weight is too low for me to reach success in the proper time frame."

This can be a problem for many people, since calf muscles, even in untrained people, are usually quite strong. Try one of these two things: Use both legs to rise up on your toes, but lower to your heels again with only one. Or exercise only one leg at a time. To do this, place your other foot behind the knee of the working leg and raise and lower on only one leg; then switch to the other side. Either method will effectively double the work your calf muscles will have to do.

"Even one-legged heel raises are too easy!"

Try going even slower than 7 seconds up, 7 down. Stretch your interval to 10, 15, or even 20 beats of the metronome. This can increase the difficulty even more.

Finis!

Congratulations! You've just completed your first Slow Burn at Home workout; if you were able to do it completely and correctly, you should feel quite fatigued and shaky, but exhilarated, and maybe even in need of a catnap. But whatever your postexercise state, you've taken an important step on your journey to strength and better health. Your first crack at following a Slow Burn regimen can be a little choppy as you become familiar with the movements and feel your way toward the right weight for each exercise. Your routine may take you longer than twenty-five to thirty minutes; that's normal and to be expected. You'll soon be able to complete it easily in that time. You'll find that each workout goes more smoothly than the last—especially if you've kept good, accurate records of what worked and what needed to be altered. Before you know it, the routine will be second nature, smooth as satin, and take you no more than a half hour from start to finish.

You should try to perform this routine at least once a week, although in the early stages, as you're getting familiar with it, you may choose to do it two or even three times a week to expedite the learning process. The ideal interval, according to medical research, is about every five days for maximum benefit. If you work hard during your routine, that twenty-five to thirty minutes every five to seven days will be all you need to make you stronger, fitter, leaner, and healthier. Once you've gotten the movements down pat and have found the correct weight for each exercise, the workout session should leave your muscles exhausted and in need of a rest period. And since Slow Burn only takes a half hour a week, you'll have more time than ever before for fun.

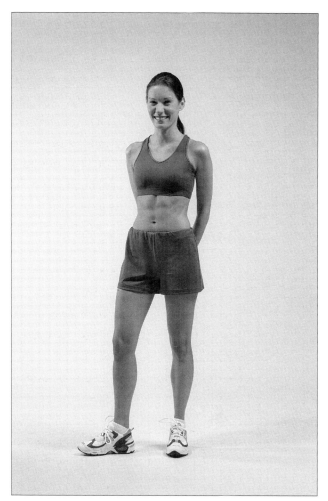

I was always a member of those large New York City gyms, doing the "same old, same old" and getting halfway decent results. Then a friend told me about Serious Strength's Slow Burn technique, and it sounded so amazing I decided to try it. Since starting the program I have never felt healthier or looked better in my entire life. The workout is incredible! My strength and endurance have skyrocketed since starting Slow Burn, and I only spend thirty minutes a week doing it. I would not go back to what I was doing for exercise before for anything.

—Katie Daily,
student, Columbia University

Slow Burn
in the Gym

CHAPTER 10

A carpenter is only as good as his tools.

—ANONYMOUS

Strength training at home can be a convenient, affordable, and private way to go about increasing your strength, improving your health, and restoring your fitness—especially as a beginner. But unless your home is outfitted with good exercise equipment, at the very least a set of barbells, dumbbells, and a weight bench, it's usually not the optimal setting for the long run. By training on machines that you can find in almost any gym or at your neighborhood fitness center or YMCA, you will reach your health and fitness goals faster and be able to more easily tailor and diversify your workout routine.

In a well-equipped gym, you'll usually find pieces of equipment that target certain muscle groups—in particular the neck and low back—that are virtually impossible to effectively work through a full range of motion using home-based techniques that rely solely on body weight or light hand and ankle weights (or milk jugs). When working at home it's also tough to progressively challenge your muscles with increasing weight as you become stronger. Soon your improved strength will outstrip the small amounts of weight we've specified in the at Home routine, and you will, at the very least, want to invest in sets of heavier weights or a set of barbells. Better yet, at that point, you may want to begin training at a well-equipped gym.

The Gym Scene

The basic rules and techniques for doing a Slow Burn workout safely and effectively stay the same whether you're in the gym or in your living room. So, to refresh yourself on the basics and for safety's sake, before you head to the gym for your first workout, go back and reread the sections in Chapter 9 entitled "Timing Is Everything," "Some Important Safety Tips Before You Begin," and "Getting with the Slow Burn Program."

While the methods don't change, the tools you'll use do. For the most part, you'll be working the same muscle groups (using machines or free weights) as you would in a home workout, plus a few additional muscle groups that just aren't possible to effectively work at home. You'll still be using your metronome, your workout progress chart and pencil, and your timer. The big difference is that you'll be working with machines in an environment that, depending on the gym, may not be as free of distractions or as quiet and conducive to focused concentration as the one you can set up at home—unless, of course, you find yourself in an authentic Slow Burn studio or other gym that provides private training only. Most gym scenes are filled with blaring TVs, thumping rock music, and the clang and clatter of improperly used weight stacks dropping with gravity. You'll have to work to blot out this clamor, but you can do it. Focus on the beat of your metronome, on your even, relaxed breathing, and on the muscle group you're working. Since you only have to do your Slow Burn routine every five to seven days, you might check with the powers that be in the gym to find out their slowest, quietest hours or days and spend your focused twenty-five to thirty minutes there at that time, when distractions will be at a minimum.

Slow Burn with Machines

Although we'd like to be able to give you specific user instructions, exact seat or pad positions, range of motion settings, and hand and foot placement positions for any machine you might encounter in whatever gym you select, their designs vary too widely for us to do so. In virtually every gym, however, there should be a qualified person on duty to help acquaint you with the machines there. So, unless you're already well versed in using the equipment at your gym, you will want to ask the advice of the trainer or instructor on site, who can help you determine the proper seat height and settings for each of the machines you will use. Often there will be placards right on the machine that can guide you on how to set it up properly. Once that's done, you'll write the settings down on your workout progress chart for future reference. Then you'll nearly be ready to use the Slow Burn technique on machines.

The only thing left to do before you can begin is to set the proper amount of weight for each exercise. You'll note that the stacks of weights all have numbers: 1 through 10, 10 through 250, 50 through 350, and so on. While it might be tempting to think that these numbers actually mean something—like weight in pounds or kilograms, for instance— the unfortunate truth is that they often don't. Different manufacturers choose different methods of marking the weight stacks on their machines, and there really isn't even a rough correlation among them. So, once again, you'll initially need to use the old trial-and-error method to get the right weight for each exercise.

How much is right? Whatever amount it takes for you to reach complete failure of the particular muscle group you're working within sixty to ninety seconds, performing between three and six repetitions. And remember, complete failure means that you cannot continue to move the weight against gravity and still maintain perfect form. If you complete a repetition, however difficult, you are obligated to try another one, even if the weight won't budge a millimeter; it's these last five to ten seconds of focused effort without result that constitute true failure. And in the Slow Burn world, failure translates into success!

The weight you select should feel relatively heavy on the first repetition; it may seem as if you can't possibly get it to move without resorting to adding momentum, but don't give in to that temptation. Just relax, breathe freely, and begin to push with a slow, steady pressure; if the weight really is too heavy, you won't even be able to budge it. Think of the kind of effort you'd apply if you had to move a stalled car. You'd get behind the car and slowly begin to push; if you kept at it, maybe the car would begin to roll. Maybe not, and then you'd simply back off, relax, and get someone to help you. What you wouldn't do is run up behind the car, jam your arms into it, and expect to get it going. You'd expect to hurt yourself if you did that. The same is true for lifting weights in the gym. If you take it slow and easy as you begin, you don't need to worry that you'll lift too heavy a weight and hurt yourself; as long as you keep the pressure steady, don't hold your breath, twist, strain, or jerk against the weight, you'll be safe. If it simply won't move despite your best, honest effort, reset the machine to the next lower weight and try again. And if necessary, lower it again and again, until you find the right setting for that exercise for you at this time.

In the beginning, you might want to choose a weight that allows for an easier first effort. This way you can learn how to do the exercises properly before encountering challenging resistance. If you choose to lighten up at first, shoot for a little longer time, 120 seconds or so; then as you become comfortable with the exercise, you can beef up the poundage and aim for fatigue within that sixty- to ninety-second span. Either method will work; it's up to you to decide whether you'd rather get the set over with sooner or have the first few repetitions be a little lighter and easier.

If the weight begins to move within the three-beat count of your metronome and feels heavy but not impossibly so, you've probably found the correct weight setting; see if you can continue to lift and lower this weight smoothly and in perfect Slow Burn form for at least sixty seconds before your muscles reach failure. If so, the weight isn't too heavy for you. If you honestly can't make the sixty-second mark before you come to complete failure, it's still a little too heavy; reduce the weight just a tiny bit next time. If, on the other hand, you're still making perfect Slow Burn inch-a-second repetitions after ninety seconds, the weight is too light for you.

For each exercise, you must determine a weight that you can lift and lower with perfect form and timing for at least sixty seconds, but ideally not more than ninety. When you've found that number, write it on your workout progress chart.

As you become stronger, you'll soon discover that this weight no longer challenges your muscles sufficiently: at the ninety-second mark your muscles haven't fatigued. If you can continue lifting the weight in perfect Slow Burn form for longer than 120 seconds and do more than a maximum of six reps, it's now time to raise the bar; you need to add more weight. Be aware that this strength adaptation won't occur simultaneously for all the exercises—each group of muscles will get stronger at its own pace.

Raising the Bar

We recommend that instead of waiting until you can continue to lift beyond six reps or longer than 120 seconds, you increase the weight for a particular machine in small increments—even as little as a pound or two—when you begin to see your progress moving toward those maximums. For instance, if you begin an exercise at a given weight and it takes you seventy-five seconds to reach failure on your fourth repetition, when you progress to the point where it takes you eighty-five or ninety seconds to reach failure on your fifth repetition, move the weight up a tiny bit. This way, you'll stay in the Slow Burn optimal success zone during every exercise period. You're aiming for this sixty-to-ninety-second zone, but adjusting the weights is an inexact science. Never lose sight of the fact that your goal is to reach success by taking your muscles to failure—not to lift a certain number of reps within an exact length of time. If during an exercise you surpass ninety seconds or 100 seconds, you shouldn't stop. You should continue to the success-through-failure endpoint for maximum benefit, having learned that this weight is insufficient and you'll need to raise it at your next session.

By making small incremental increases—a technique called microloading—you can make amazing gains in strength without ever feeling it. For example, suppose you begin by properly lifting 100 pounds on a particular machine. If once a week in your Slow Burn session you can make a mere 1-pound increase in the weight you're lifting, by the end of a year, you'll be lifting 152 pounds—that's more than a 50 percent increase in your strength.

Or instead, you might want to adopt a stair-stepped progression technique in which you make the increases in larger periodic jumps as you reach your target in duration or repetitions. The general rule here is to increase the weight by 5 percent when you begin to near your target maximums. Again, since it's hard to know exactly how much weight you're lifting on some machines because the weight stacks aren't measured in pounds, you may have to do some estimating. Fortunately, the weights on most machines increase in set increments of five, ten, or twenty units from one plate to the next.

Often, the machines will also have add-on weights, or saddle plates, that sit securely on the weight stacks, allowing you to make smaller adjustments.

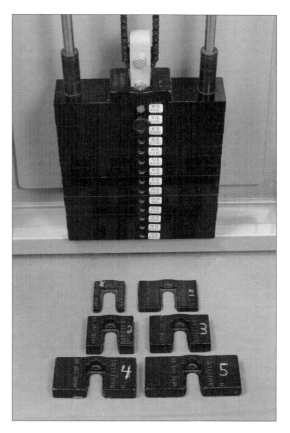

These additional weights may come in increments ranging from half a pound to as much as ten pounds; however, many gyms have only five- or ten-pound add-on (or saddle) plates. If this is the case in your gym and you need to make a smaller incremental increase, you can use a 1¼-, 2½-, or 5-pound round free-weight plate that you can "pin" through onto the weight stack. Although these methods will work, they can also be a bit hazardous, since the weights could slip and fall off. It's a better idea, if possible, to try nudging your gym manager into purchasing a few inexpensive saddle plates for the facility.

By whatever means you choose to make your increases, be aware that if you're out of condition when you join the Slow Burn Fitness Revolution, your strength gains will at first be quite dramatic. From one week to the next, you can almost feel your strength building, and you'll find that you need to increase weight regularly. Once you've become stronger and better conditioned, however, you'll see the skyrocketing trajectory of improvement begin to level off to a somewhat steadier and more deliberate pace. The increases will be smaller and perhaps not as frequent.

A word of caution: If you experience joint pain as you work through the range of motion of any exercise using machines, you can limit the excursion of the machine by pinning off the weight stack. Simply lift the weight arm up (or push it down, depending on the machine) and put a weight stack pin into the hole on the stack to effectively shorten the range of motion through which you'll push the weight.

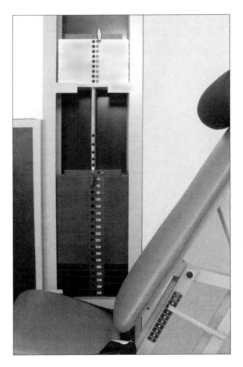

FULL RANGE OF MOTION

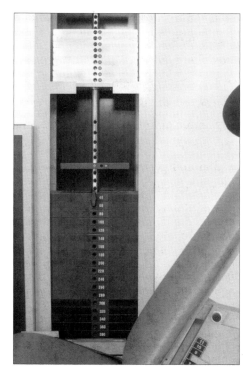

PARTIAL RANGE OF MOTION, WITH WEIGHT
PINNED

Let's take a look now at the exercises you'll want to do in the gym.

The Slow Burn Gym Routine

Although you'll see thirteen exercises described, we would recommend that you select six or seven of them at first—depending on the availability of machines in your gym—and perform them *in the exact order given.* As you get the hang of it, you can add a few more, building to a total of nine or ten, or all thirteen. (Note, however, that as you become stronger and stronger and your weekly routine becomes more challenging, you will probably want to revert to the six to eight main exercises you started with. If you try to do all thirteen exercises in a row, you may find yourself becoming so fatigued that your form and concentration fade, and that could lead to an injury.) If you'd like to do them all, that's dandy, but don't try to do it in one routine. Instead, create two different routines for yourself—for example, a Routine A that includes exercises 1, 2, 4, 5, 7, 10, and 13 and a Routine B that includes exercises 3, 6, 8, 9, 11, and 12—and alternate the routines in successive workouts. If you choose to adopt the dual-routine regimen, you should probably not space your workout sessions further apart than every five days. In our opinion two shorter sessions per week are better than one long one, but everyone's time constraints are different; it's sufficient to be consistent about doing at least one session per week. Some people prefer to do three very short sessions per week, and this seems to work well also. It's up to you to decide. These are the general rules of the Slow Burn workout for any of the exercises:

- Complete all repetitions in perfect form; never strain, twist, arch your back, crane your neck, slouch, or "jerk" or "drop" the weight to complete a repetition. Remember, the true objective is to reach the deepest level of fatigue possible in the target muscle(s), not to complete a certain number of reps in any way you can.
- Never hold your breath; always breathe in a relaxed, even fashion throughout the exercise.
- Try to keep a neutral, focused attitude during the exercise; never clench your teeth or grimace.
- Always work through a full, pain-free range of joint motion.
- Remember your timing: 3/7/3/7. Take three full beats to begin to move the weight the first inch; execute a smooth,

slow lift, moving the weight at a pace of about one inch per second (a minimum of seven beats of the metronome to complete the lift); make a very slow reversal of direction, taking three beats to complete the change; finish the repetition just as slowly, moving the weight about one inch per second on its return to the starting position.

Because your safety must always come first, along with this list of exercises for doing the Slow Burn in the Gym, you'll find some important Do's and Don'ts specific to each one. Take them to heart.

#1 Neck Extension[*]

Works the muscles of the back of the neck (cervical extensors)

Do:

- Sit up tall, elongate your neck, and drop your shoulders to a relaxed position
- Keep your lips closed, in this instance, but your jaw relaxed. In doing so you will give a nice stretch to your frontal neck muscles.
- Keep your head facing forward
- Press the back of your head against the pad, thinking of going first straight back, then straight down as if making an L shape instead of an arc. Do the same coming forward.

Don't:

- Slouch, lean forward or backward, sway from side to side, or shrug your shoulders
- Jut out your jaw, clench your teeth, or grimace
- Twist or turn your head from side to side

The Technique:

- From Start position, take three full seconds to move the first inch.
- Moving as smoothly as possible, take a minimum of seven seconds (longer is fine, too) to raise the weight to the Finish position, moving no faster than one inch per second.
- Take three full seconds to reverse direction for the first inch out of Finish position.
- Then take a minimum of seven seconds to lower the weight back to Start.
- Repeat this cycle until no further repetitions are possible in perfect form.

Many gyms do not have a neck extension machine or a lower-back machine; check Appendix A for a list of gyms that have them. Be aware that without such machines, it's very difficult to isolate the muscles of these areas, work them to failure, and strengthen them. See Chapter 7 to learn more about the benefits of directly working the neck and low back.

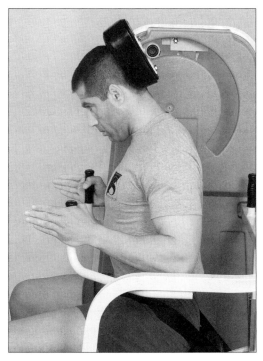

START

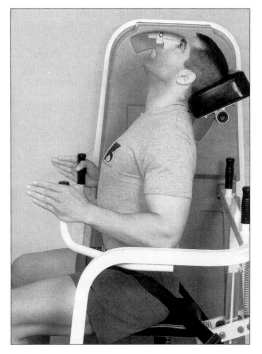

FINISH

#2 Chest Press

Works the muscles of the chest (the "pecs"), as well as the muscles of the arms (triceps) and shoulders (front deltoids)

Do:

- Keep your shoulders down
- Keep your chin slightly tucked and your neck elongated
- Keep your chest "proud" and upright
- Keep your elbows at a 45-degree angle from your sides
- Keep a slight bend in your elbows at the finish point
- Keep your hands in line with your armpits at the start
- Keep your lower back slightly arched throughout
- Keep your hands loose around the grip(s)

Don't:

- Shrug your shoulders
- Crane your neck or tip your head back with your chin up
- Slouch or let your chest "cave in"
- Lock your elbows at the finish point
- Let your hands and arms rise above the level of your shoulders or drop below your rib cage
- Arch suddenly to finish a repetition
- Grip the handles or bar tightly

The Technique:

- From Start position, take three full seconds to move the first inch.
- Moving as smoothly as possible, take a minimum of seven seconds (longer is fine, too) to raise the weight to the Finish position, moving no faster than one inch per second.
- Take three full seconds to reverse direction for the first inch out of Finish position.
- Then take a minimum of seven seconds to lower the weight back to Start.
- Repeat this cycle until no further repetitions are possible in perfect form.

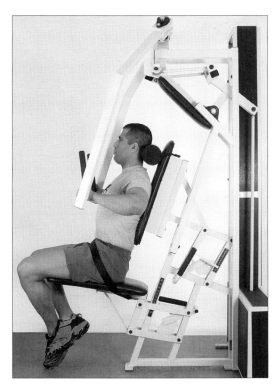

START

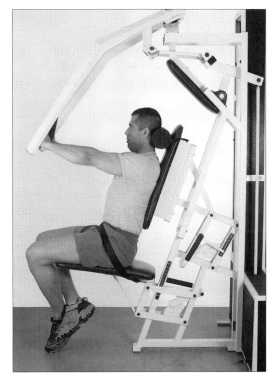

FINISH

#3 Knee Flexion

Works the muscles of the back of the thighs (hamstrings) and the calves

Do:

- Align your knee joint with the machine's axis of rotation (ask the on-site expert to check your position if you're unsure)
- Keep your kneecaps facing the ceiling and your legs parallel and evenly spaced
- Keep your toes flexed toward you as if they were reaching for your knees
- Let your back arch naturally

Don't:

- Attempt the exercise with your knee joint in front of or behind the machine's axis of rotation
- Spread your ankles apart
- Point your toes
- Suddenly arch your back

The Technique:

- From Start position, take three full seconds to move the first inch.
- Moving as smoothly as possible, take a minimum of seven seconds (longer is fine, too) to raise the weight to the Finish position, moving no faster than one inch per second.
- Take three full seconds to reverse direction for the first inch out of Finish position.
- Then take a minimum of seven seconds to lower the weight back to Start.
- Repeat this cycle until no further repetitions are possible in perfect form.

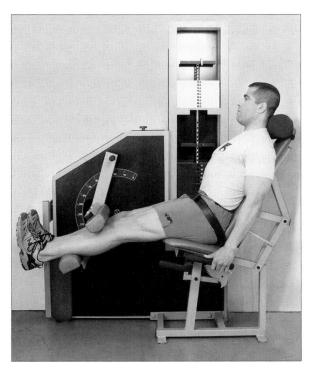

START

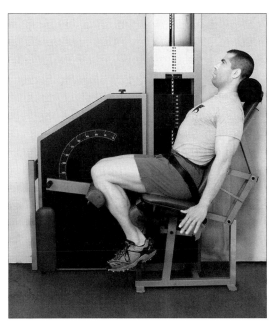

FINISH

#4 Leg Press

Works the buttocks ("glutes") and the muscles of both the front and back of the thighs ("quads" and hamstrings)

Do:
- Keep your knees slightly bent at the endpoint
- Keep your hands loose at your sides
- Keep your legs parallel to each other, your knees and toes aligned, and your feet spaced a hip's width apart

Don't:
- Lock your knees
- Grip the handles tightly or put your hands on your thighs to push
- Let your knees knock or your feet turn out

The Technique:
- From Start position, take three full seconds to move the first inch.
- Moving as smoothly as possible, take a minimum of seven seconds (longer is fine, too) to raise the weight to the Finish position, moving no faster than one inch per second.
- Take three full seconds to reverse direction for the first inch out of Finish position.
- Then take a minimum of seven seconds to lower the weight back to Start.
- Repeat this cycle until no further repetitions are possible in perfect form.

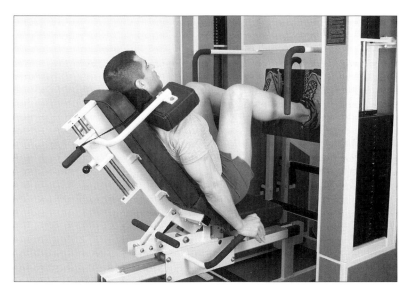

Start

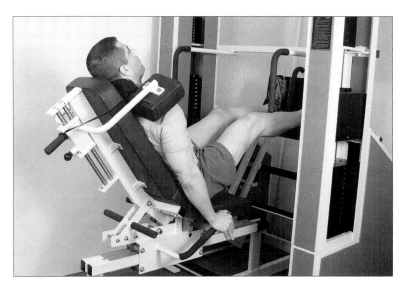

Finish

#5 Hip Adduction

Works the inner thighs and the hip muscles (hip adductors, the horseback-riding muscles)

Do:

- Keep your knees straight
- Keep your thighs straight and your kneecaps and toes pointed toward the ceiling

Don't:

- Let your knees bend
- Let your thighs, knees, and toes rotate outward

The Technique:

- From Start position, take three full seconds to move the first inch.
- Moving as smoothly as possible, take a minimum of seven seconds (longer is fine, too) to raise the weight to the Finish position, moving no faster than one inch per second.
- Take three full seconds to reverse direction for the first inch out of Finish position.
- Then take a minimum of seven seconds to lower the weight back to Start.
- Repeat this cycle until no further repetitions are possible in perfect form.

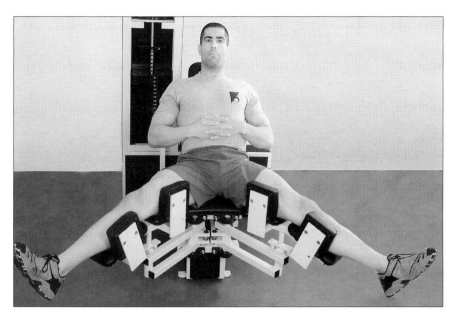

Start

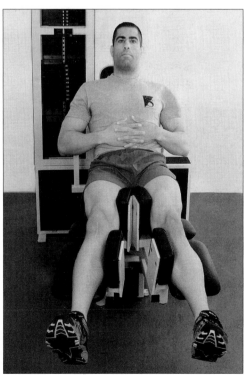

Finish

#6 Back Pulldowns
(Lat Pulldowns)

Works the muscles of the back ("lats"), the muscles of the front and back of the arms (biceps and triceps), and the muscles of the forearms

Do:

- Use a "palms-facing-you" grip
- Place your hands a shoulder's width apart
- Keep a slight bend in the elbows when starting

Don't:

- Use a "palms-away-from-you" grip
- Position your hands too close together or too far apart
- Allow your elbows to "lock" straight in extension

The Technique:

- From Start position, take three full seconds to move the first inch.
- Moving as smoothly as possible, take a minimum of seven seconds (longer is fine, too) to raise the weight to the Finish position, moving no faster than one inch per second.
- Take three full seconds to reverse direction for the first inch out of Finish position.
- Then take a minimum of seven seconds to lower the weight back to Start.
- Repeat this cycle until no further repetitions are possible in perfect form.

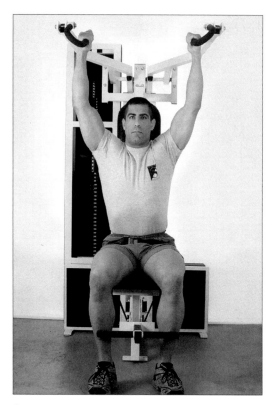

START

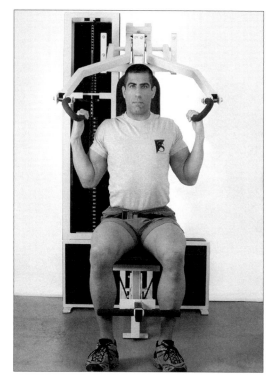

FINISH

#7 Shoulder Side Raises

Works the muscles of the shoulders (deltoids and trapezoids)

Do:
- Keep your back snugly against the back pad
- Pause at the point where your arms are parallel to the ground or slightly above parallel

Don't:
- Lean forward or arch your back excessively
- Raise your elbows and arms above shoulder height

The Technique:
- From Start position, take three full seconds to move the first inch.
- Moving as smoothly as possible, take a minimum of seven seconds (longer is fine, too) to raise the weight to the Finish position, moving no faster than one inch per second.
- Take three full seconds to reverse direction for the first inch out of Finish position.
- Then take a minimum of seven seconds to lower the weight back to Start.
- Repeat this cycle until no further repetitions are possible in perfect form.

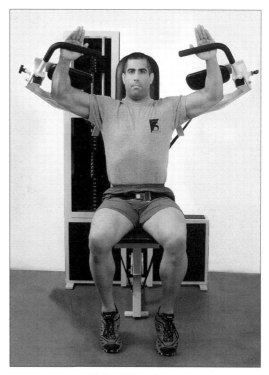

FINISH

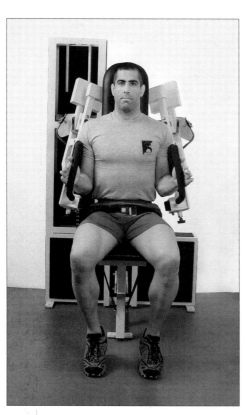

START

#8 Overhead Shoulder Press

Works the shoulders (deltoids) and the muscles of the backs of the arms (triceps)

Do:
- Keep your hands slightly in front of your shoulders
- Keep your back flat (against the back pad if there is one) with good upright posture and a "proud" chest

Don't:
- Position your hands beside or behind your shoulders
- Slouch down or "cave" your chest
- Violently arch your back
- Grip your hands too tightly

The Technique:
- From Start position, take three full seconds to move the first inch.
- Moving as smoothly as possible, take a minimum of seven seconds (longer is fine, too) to raise the weight to the Finish position, moving no faster than one inch per second.
- Take three full seconds to reverse direction for the first inch out of Finish position.
- Then take a minimum of seven seconds to lower the weight back to Start.
- Repeat this cycle until no further repetitions are possible in perfect form.

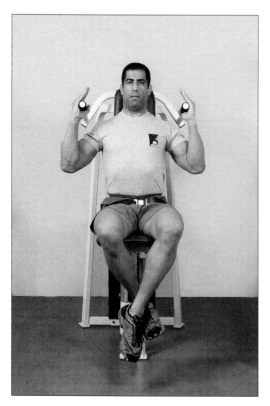

Start

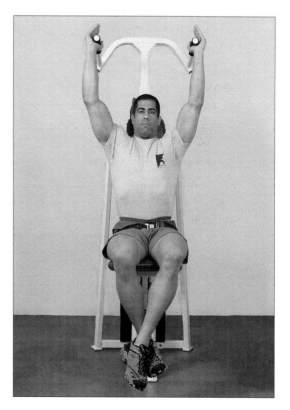

Finish

#9 Rowing Back (or Rowing torso)

Works the muscles of the upper back and shoulders (trapezius, rhomboids, rear deltoids)

Do:

- Sit up tall, keeping your shoulders down
- Press the pads away using your forearm and elbows
- Keep your arms parallel to the ground

Don't:

- Shrug your shoulders
- Push with your hands
- Lurch backward
- Raise or lower your elbows

The Technique:

- From Start position, take three full seconds to move the first inch.
- Moving as smoothly as possible, take a minimum of seven seconds (longer is fine, too) to raise the weight to the Finish position, moving no faster than one inch per second.
- Take three full seconds to reverse direction for the first inch out of Finish position.
- Then take a minimum of seven seconds to lower the weight back to Start.
- Repeat this cycle until no further repetitions are possible in perfect form.

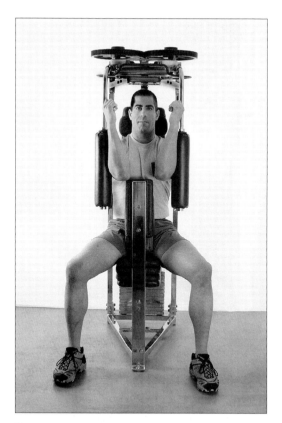

Start

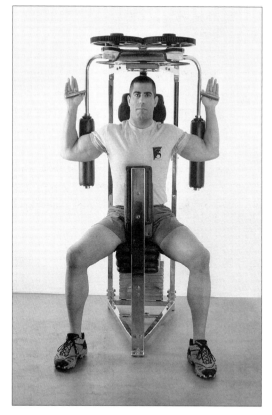

Finish

#10 Biceps Curl

Works the muscles at the front of the upper arm (biceps) and the muscles of the fore-arm

Do:

- Keep your shoulders down
- Keep your elbows slightly bent at extension
- Keep your elbows and upper arms "glued" to your sides

Don't:

- Shrug or hunch your shoulders
- Allow your elbows to fully straighten or "lock" at extension
- Allow your upper arms and elbows to drift away from your sides

The Technique:

- From Start position, take three full seconds to move the first inch.
- Moving as smoothly as possible, take a minimum of seven seconds (longer is fine, too) to raise the weight to the Finish position, moving no faster than one inch per second.
- Take three full seconds to reverse direction for the first inch out of Finish position.
- Then take a minimum of seven seconds to lower the weight back to Start.
- Repeat this cycle until no further repetitions are possible in perfect form.

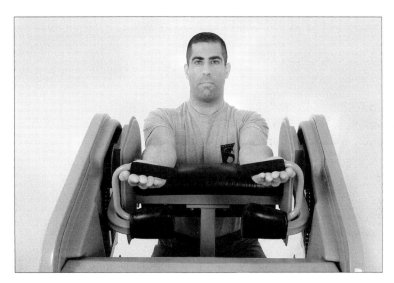

START

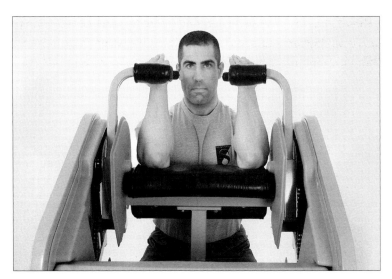

FINISH

#11 Abdominal Crunches

Works the stomach muscles, or "abs"

Do:

- Keep your head and neck straight and relaxed
- Flex your spine and curl your trunk

Don't:

- Flex or extend your neck
- Pivot forward from your hips

The Technique:

- From Start position, take three full seconds to move the first inch.
- Moving as smoothly as possible, take a minimum of seven seconds (longer is fine, too) to raise the weight to the Finish position, moving no faster than one inch per second.
- Take three full seconds to reverse direction for the first inch out of Finish position.
- Then take a minimum of seven seconds to lower the weight back to Start.
- Repeat this cycle until no further repetitions are possible in perfect form.

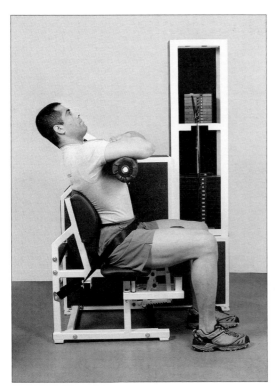

Start

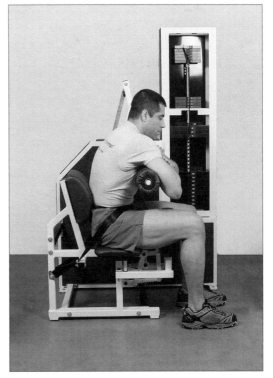

Finish

#12 Lower Back Extension*

Works the muscles of the very low back (lumbar area)

Do:
- Use the seat belt to keep your pelvis still
- Sit up tall and straight at the start
- Lean backward in a smooth, straight line
- Arch your back fully as you come forward at the finish

Don't:
- Allow yourself to pivot from your hips or you won't be working your back
- Twist or shift from side to side as you lean back
- Slouch in the finish

The Technique:
- From Start position, take three full seconds to move the first inch.
- Moving as smoothly as possible, take a minimum of seven seconds (longer is fine, too) to raise the weight to the Finish position, moving no faster than one inch per second.
- Take three full seconds to reverse direction for the first inch out of Finish position.
- Then take a minimum of seven seconds to lower the weight back to Start.
- Repeat this cycle until no further repetitions are possible in perfect form.

Many gyms do not have a neck extension machine or a lower-back machine; check Appendix A for a list of gyms that have them. Be aware that without such machines, it's very difficult to isolate the muscles of these areas, work them to failure, and strengthen them. See Chapter 7 to learn more about the benefits of directly working the neck and low back.

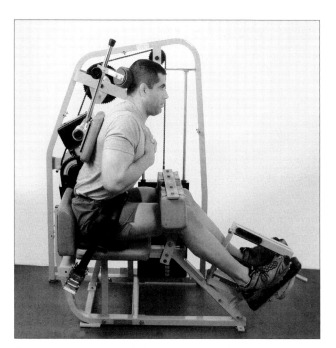

START

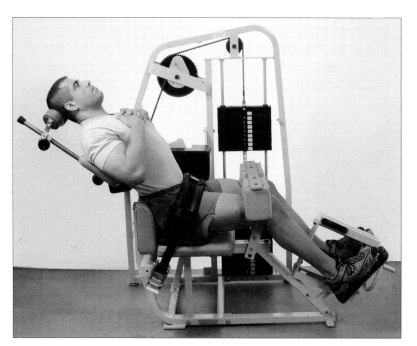

FINISH

#13 Heel Raises (Calf Raises)

Works the muscles of the lower legs (calves)

Do:

- Keep your feet parallel
- Press mainly with your big toe and its nearest two neighbors
- Pivot on the balls of your feet

Don't:

- Let your heels turn inward or outward
- Let your feet roll outward onto your "pinky" toes
- Pivot on the arches of your feet

The Technique:

- From Start position, take three full seconds to move the first inch.
- Moving as smoothly as possible, take a minimum of seven seconds (longer is fine, too) to raise the weight to the Finish position, moving no faster than one inch per second.
- Take three full seconds to reverse direction for the first inch out of Finish position.
- Then take a minimum of seven seconds to lower the weight back to Start.
- Repeat this cycle until no further repetitions are possible in perfect form.

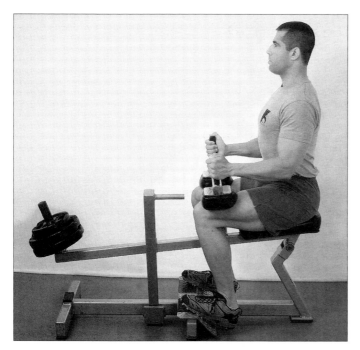

START

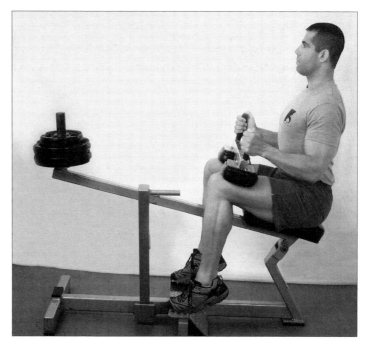

FINISH

Finis!

So you've now completed your first Slow Burn in the Gym session. You may feel a bit of fatigue now, but you'll be amazed at how quickly you recover. And you'll be surprised at how little residual soreness you feel in the morning after a Slow Burn workout, compared to other methods of strength training. That's yet another virtue of the Slow Burn technique—lifting slowly for a few reps works the muscles but doesn't cause jolting repetitive trauma to the joints that leaves you hobbling about in misery the next day and the day after that.

You should also feel quite exhilarated, since you've taken the first step on your journey to a leaner, stronger, fitter, and healthier you. Welcome to the Slow Burn Revolution!

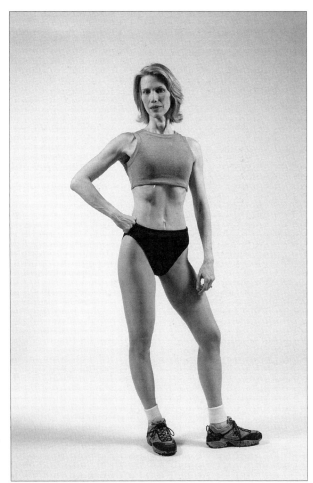

In 1997 I met Fred Hahn, who introduced me to Slow Burn strength training. I cut out all aerobic exercise and did Slow Burn exclusively. After a couple months, I noticed subtle changes. People who hadn't seen me in a while said I looked as though I had lost ten pounds.

My body-fat percentage now is 4 percent less than it was when I was doing hours a week of so-called "fat-burning" aerobics. I no longer have the kind of overuse injuries that many people my age begin to complain about. I am in better overall condition at the age of forty-eight than I was twenty years ago. I wish I had known then what I know now!

—Lisa C. Feldman

Resource List

Any local sports store will have the very basic equipment you need to get started doing the Slow Burn home routine. As noted earlier, you can even make weights out of materials you already have in your kitchen. But in case you want to treat yourself to the best equipment, here is a list of various companies that will aid you in your search for either gym or home exercise equipment, including saddle plates (also called fractional plates), dumbbells, ankle weights, benches, and a variety of other items you can use to bolster your strength and fitness.

The Gym Source	www.gymsource.com
Ironmind Enterprises	www.ironmind.com
MedX	www.medxonline.com
Nautilus	www.nautilus.com
Piedmont Design Associates	www.fractionalplates.com

The following fitness centers and instructors provide expert instruction in exercise systems similar to Slow Burn. The website for Fred Hahn's fitness center, Serious Strength, is www.seriousstrength.com

Belmar Intelligent Exercise Belmar, New Jersey	www.belmar-fitness.com
Intelligent Exercise Shreveport, Louisiana	www.ieshreveport.com
Maxercise Philadelphia, Pennsylvania	www.maxercise.com
The New York Exercise Company Brooklyn, New York	www.newyorkexercise.com
Precision Fitness Naperville, Illinois	www.precisionfitnessinc.com

Please visit our website www.seriousstrength.com for other health and fitness links. We offer a rich resource of information designed to help you understand the philosophy and benefits of Slow Burn and become the healthiest you can be. We update the site frequently, so check back often!

For a free sample issue of the *Eades Health Report* newsletter, write to Editor, Eades Health Report, P.O. Box 62, Denver, CO 80201 or visit www.eadeshealthreport.com, where you'll find up-to-date nutritional and health information. Also visit the Drs. Eadeses' site at www.eatprotein.com for information on available nutritional products or for dietary support.

The Slow Burn Progress Chart

The Slow Burn Progress Chart will allow you to track your session-by-session progress. It will also help you organize the practical details of your workouts, such as the machine settings that you use if you work out at a gym. Make several photocopies of the blank chart on page 172 and use it every time you do Slow Burn.

SAMPLE ENTRY:

THE **SLOW BURN** PROGRESS CHART		Date: _9/27_ Body Weight: _136_ Daily Notes: _Felt great start-ing. Slept really well last night._		
Name of Exercise	**Machine Settings**	**Weight/ Order**	**Time to Failure/ Reps Completed**	
Chest Press	Back 3 Seat 6	100 / 1	1:26 / 5	

At the top of the chart you'll note the *Date* and your *Body Weight.* You'll also have room in the *Daily Notes* space for taking note of any factors that may affect your workout, such as having a cold or feeling particularly good. Don't neglect this aspect of the Slow Burn Progress Chart. Over time it will help you remember certain issues that may become important later on.

Machine Settings: This box is for those using the gym program. Here you will record the settings you use to adapt each machine to your height and size. Most machines use numbers to mark the various seat heights or back pad settings. Once you've learned the right settings for you, you will probably not have to change them. Ask your local gym expert to show you how to mark the particular settings for the machines at your gym.

Weight: This is where you record the weight you use.

Order: Here you record the order in which you did the exercises that day. You should try to do the exercises in the order specified in the text, but that may not always be possible (for example, if there is a long wait for a certain machine).

Time to Failure: Record in minutes and seconds the length of time it took you to push your muscles to the success-through-failure endpoint.

Repetitions Completed: Here you'll record the number of *complete* repetitions you were able to perform for that exercise.

THE SLOW BURN PROGRESS CHART

Name of Exercise	Machine Settings	Date: _____ Body Weight: _____ Daily Notes:		Date: _____ Body Weight: _____ Daily Notes:		Date: _____ Body Weight: _____ Daily Notes:	
		Weight/ Order	Time to Failure/ Reps Completed	Weight/ Order	Time to Failure/ Reps Completed	Weight/ Order	Time to Failure/ Reps Completed

The Slow Burn Power Eating Plan

There's no more effective tool to lose excess body fat and build your lean body mass than a diet rich in protein, adequate in good quality fats and oils, filled with fresh fruits and colorful vegetables, but restricted in starches and sugars. To help you reach your health and fitness goals with the Slow Burn Fitness Revolution, we've provided lists of the kinds of foods for a healthy diet as well as a week of meal plans to help you get started.

In general, we recommend that to correct weight or health issues using a low-carb diet, you must first be sure to eat adequate protein at each meal and keep carbohydrates restricted to 10 to 15 grams of effective carbohydrate (i.e., absorbable sugar and starch) per meal or snack. Your meal plans are scaled to give you about that amount. Subsequently, you can add more carbohydrate-containing foods from the lists that follow.[1]

Select from these mainly protein foods:

[1] See our books *Protein Power* (New York: Bantam, 1996) or *The Protein Power Lifeplan* (New York: Warner, 2000) for complete details.

At breakfast:

Eggs, any style (with meat, cheese, or fish, if desired); om-
lets (with meat, cheese, or fish, if desired); protein shakes;
cottage cheese

At lunch or dinner:

Hamburger, steak, roast beef, chicken, turkey, ham, pork,
kielbasa or Italian sausage, veal, tuna, salmon, swordfish,
sardines, mackerel, herring, lobster, shrimp, scallops, cala-
mari, clams, oysters, freshwater fish, chicken salad, tuna
salad, egg salad, tofu, veggie burgers

All meat, poultry, and fish should be grilled, poached,
sautéed, braised, or boiled—never breaded and fried.[2]

To accompany your protein choice, select from these fruits
and vegetables—all mainly carbohydrate foods:

Vegetables

Artichokes, asparagus, aubergine, bamboo shoots, beets,
broccoli, Brussels sprouts, cabbage, carrots, cauliflower, celery, chard, coleslaw, cucumber, fennel, greens, green beans,
kale, kelp, leeks, lettuces, mushrooms, okra, onions, green
peas, peppers, pimientos, radicchio, rhubarb, rutabaga,
sauerkraut, shallots, spinach, summer and winter squashes,
tomato, turnips, and water chestnuts

[2]The only permissible way to bread and fry meat, poultry, and fish can
be found in our new *Low-Carb Comfort Food Cookbook*, which contains
over 300 recipes for low-carb comfort delights useful to you on your Slow
Burn regimen, including breads, muffins, waffles, pies, cakes, cookies,
pizza, tortillas, and pasta. Available at bookstores nationwide.

As with meat, fish, and poultry, all vegetables should be boiled, poached, grilled, sautéed, or eaten raw—never breaded and fried.

Fruits

Apple (small), avocado, banana (½ small), blackberries, blueberries, cantaloupe, cherries, currants, grapefruit, grapes, guava, honeydew, kiwi, lemon, lime, nectarine, orange, passion fruit, peach (small), pear (small), pineapple, raspberries, strawberries, tangerine, watermelon

Eat the fruits fresh, frozen without sugar, or canned without sugar or syrup.

Dairy

Dairy products such as cheese, cream, and yogurt are also permissible, but these foods contain both carbohydrate as well as protein. The same is true for nuts and seeds. In hard cheeses, cream, nuts, and seeds there's not much carbohydrate, but in fluid dairy products there's about 1 to 1½ grams of carbohydrate in every ounce. If you are trying to lose weight, overeating dairy products, nuts, or nut butters can stall your progress.

We encourage you to drink at least 64 ounces of noncaloric fluid (water, herbal tea, decaf coffee) each day and to take some extra potassium and magnesium, as well as a good multivitamin and mineral supplement.[3]

[3]For complete details on vitamin and mineral supplementation, as well as the full how-to of doing a low-carb diet, pick up a copy of *Protein Power* (New York: Bantam, 1996) or *The Protein Power LifePlan* (Warner 2000).

Fats and Oils

Quality is essential. Choose from butter, olive oil, nut oils, and coconut oil. Avoid partially hydrogenated vegetable oils (such as corn, safflower, soybean, sunflower, canola), margarine, and vegetable shortening.

A week of meal plans

Day 1

Breakfast:
Scrambled eggs, sugarless ham
½ to 1 cup blueberries with 2 tablespoons cream

Lunch:
Chicken salad on a bed of lettuce
Tomato wedges (1 medium tomato)
Vinaigrette dressing

Dinner:
Grilled steak
Green salad with dressing
½ to 1 cup carrots cooked with butter

Snack:
2 to 3 celery stalks with
1 to 2 tablespoons peanut butter

Day 2

Breakfast:
Omelet with broccoli, diced tomato, and cheese
½ to 1 cup fresh strawberries

Lunch:
Grilled chicken Caesar salad
1 small tangerine

Dinner:
Grilled chicken breast
1 cup broccoli cooked with butter
½ cup berries (dollop of whipped cream, if desired)

Snack:
Macadamia nuts or peanuts

DAY 3

Breakfast:
1 to 2 slices low-carb bread, topped with melted cheese and Canadian bacon
½ to 1 cup melon

Lunch:
Ham salad on a bed of lettuce
½ fresh apple

Dinner:
Grilled salmon (or other fish)
½ cup courgettes
Fresh spinach salad with vinaigrette dressing
½ sliced apple

Snack:
Deviled egg halves

DAY 4

Breakfast:
Cottage cheese topped with fresh or frozen fruit (orange slices, berries, melon)

Lunch:
Turkey, bacon, cheese wrap (on a low-carb tortilla⁴) with lettuce, diced tomatoes, mayo, mustard, and pickle
½ orange or tangerine

⁴You can find fat-free, whole-wheat, low-carb tortillas at La Tortilla Factory at www.latortillafactory.com.

Dinner:
Roast beef or pork
Grilled tomato halves (brushed with olive oil)
Green salad with vinaigrette, ranch, or blue cheese dressing

Snack:
String cheese and 1 small apple

DAY 5

Breakfast:
Eggs any style
Sausage link
½ grapefruit

Lunch:
Tuna salad wrap (on a low-carb tortilla) with lettuce, diced tomato, mayo (if desired)
½ cup grapes

Dinner:
Taco salad without shell on a bed of lettuce
Guacamole
½ apple or pear

Snack:
Deli meat slices
Fresh cauliflower with ranch dressing

DAY 6

Breakfast:
Scrambled egg and cheese burrito (on a low-carb tortilla)
Bacon or sausage
½ to 1 cup fresh or frozen berries

Lunch:
Cheeseburger without bun (wrapped in 2 large lettuce leaves)
1 tangerine

Dinner:
Baked chicken
1 cup green beans
Tomato slices with dressing (1 medium tomato)

Snack:
½ apple with cheddar cheese

DAY 7

Breakfast:
Eggs Benedict without muffin
on a bed of steamed spinach
½ to 1 cup fresh or frozen berries

Lunch:
Grilled turkey and cheese sandwich
(open-faced on low-carb bread)
Green salad with dressing
1 small tangerine

Dinner:
Spareribs
Grilled portabello mushroom cap and sliced peppers
Green salad with dressing

Snack:
Plain yogurt and strawberries

Acknowledgments

Every book is a collaboration of the efforts of many people, but, in this instance, a true collaboration existed. We wish to acknowledge our coauthor, Fred Hahn, for introducing us to Slow Burn training, which has changed our lives.

In addition, this work would never have found its home at Broadway without our ever-faithful, hard-working agents, Channa Taub and Carol Mann. Our deepest thanks to them and to the good people at Broadway Books (especially our editor Kris Puopolo) for making this book a reality.

Thanks go as well to our colleagues Loren Cordain, Ph.D. and Larry McCleary, M.D., for tirelessly helping us locate needed research on a moment's notice and for being sounding boards for us as we unearthed the science that underlies Slow Burn.

A special thanks goes to our indispensable assistants: our muse, Debbi Judd, and Kristi McAfee, who always makes herself available to help us in any way at ungodly hours and on her days off—and even on her vacation. We couldn't have done it without you, KB.

And last, as always, our thanks and our love go to our sons, daughters-in-law, and grandsons for whom we do all we do.

—Michael R. Eades, M.D. and Mary Dan Eades, M.D.

The following people made this book possible:

Danny Dray, a kid from grade school who put the first barbell in my hand;

Dr. Ellington Darden, whose books on exercise started me thinking logically about exercise;

Arthur Jones, creator of Nautilus and MedX exercise equipment who helped pioneer the fitness industry out of the Stone Age;

Ken Hutchins, for his Super Slow technical manual that helped me become a better technical instructor;

Dr. Ben Bocchiccio, Dr. Ralph Carpinelli, Dr. Richard Winett, Matt Bryzcki, whose conversations on exercise have helped me greatly;

Tim Ryan, expert instructor and friend who influences my ideas on exercise all the time;

Peter Cohen, best friend and my training partner since high school;

Erna Miciunas, Loretta and George Lenko, my in-laws, who lent us the money to start Serious Strength;

And *most* importantly to my wife, Linda, who, as I wrote volumes of articles on exercise over the years, taught me the difference between a noun and a verb and whose confidence in me and love for me made this book truly possible.

—Fred Hahn

About the Authors

A professional exercise trainer for over twenty years, FRED HAHN founded Serious Strength, Inc., in 1998. Certified by the American Council on Exercise, he is president and co-founder of the National Council for Exercise Standards. He lives in New York City with his wife, Linda, and daughters Georgia and Amber. You can learn more about him and his strength-training program at www.seriousstrength.com.

MICHAEL R. EADES, M.D., and MARY DAN EADES, M.D. wrote the *New York Times* bestseller *Protein Power* as well as *The Protein Power Lifeplan, The Protein Power Lifeplan Gram Counter*, and *The Low-Carb Comfort Food Cookbook*. They have practiced metabolic medicine for nearly twenty years and are now on the adjunct faculty of the Department of Health and Exercise Science at Colorado State University. They divide their time between Santa Fe, New Mexico, and Incline Village, Nevada.